"Willie Johnson has penned a wonderfully-inspired book based both on his mastery of kung-fu and his rise from a street kid to prominence in the world of martial arts. This book is about much more than martial arts. Grand Master Johnson has evolved beyond physical technique into the world of personal spirituality. He presents a journey well worth reading."

—Dr. Jerry Beasley, PhD, 8th dan, author, professor of Health and
Human Performance at Radford University

"I have known Sifu Johnson for over twenty years and was an admirer of his incredible skill as a competitor in the early 90s. My first introduction to him was when I was the promoter for my father's tournament in Washington, DC (The Jhoon Rhee Nationals). What is even more impressive about him is his incredible heart and how much he cares for the people in his community. It is common knowledge that he had a rough past, but he has owned up to it and his experience with this difficult time in his life has transformed him into an amazing human being. Sifu Johnson is one of the very few martial artists that I can confidently say "walks the talk." He is an inspiring and motivational instructor and has a wealth of knowledge with respect to street self-defense. I highly recommend this book to all people regardless of their level of skill in the martial arts."

—Master Chun Rhee, owner Jhoon Rhee Tae Kwon Do,
Nobody Bothers Me, Inc., Falls Church, VA

"This book was a joy to read. I was intrigued by 'The Bam's' most recent book as it depicts how one can use martial arts to help focus on traditional core values as well as the physical and mental benefits that also result. In addition, the fact that self-defense is also highlighted in this book makes it a book that not only challenges its readers to become health conscientious but also prepares them for whatever comes their way. This book is much more than simply a focus on martial arts. This book aims to challenge and promote the mind, body, and soul in each of us."

—Dr. Lance Stout, Deputy Superintendent of Schools, Independence, Missouri,
PhD in Doctor of Education in Educational Leadership, Wichita State University

"This book is a gift to the world from a man who lays bare his heart and his struggles in the hope of bringing positive effect on the people it touches. His dedication as a martial artist is only matched by his dedication to do the hard work in local communities to show people a better path to a fulfilling life. Do yourself a favor and share this book and Willie 'The Bam' Johnson's philosophy with those around you. We'll all be better for it."

—Matt Dean, film and TV Producer, Los Angeles

"Willie Bam Johnson's extraordinary ability to share his life experiences and life lessons in compelling speeches and talks that are full of powerful insights make him a very dynamic and charismatic speaker. He has a unique ability to connect with both the youth and their parents."

—Warrington Hudlin, film and TV Producer, New York

"Seeing the challenges that Willie 'The Bam' Johnson faced at every turn in life, and his overcoming of one hardship after another through the discipline of Martial Arts will make you put yourself back on the floor with renewed dedication to the path of a better life."

—Kris Wilder, author, U.S. Martial Arts Hall of Fame member,
National Board-Certified Life Coach

"Willie 'The Bam' Johnson shares highs and lows from his life, and how these events taught him and shaped the philosophy he shares in *The Complete Martial Artist*. The lessons learned from these significant life events are universal and they can be applied by any martial artist, regardless of style or rank. Johnson's *wushudo* will help you along your road of self-development. With a focus on developing physical, mental, and spiritual fitness, the twelve universal principles of *wushudo* will not only help you become a better martial artist, but a better person through training in the martial arts. Many martial artists teach that martial arts provide a road toward not only self-defense, but also fitness, character development, and spirit. Willie Johnson provides you a map to do just that, develop yourself physically, mentally, and spiritually."

—Alain Burrese, J.D., former army sniper, 5th dan Hapkido,
author of *Hard-Won Wisdom From The School Of Hard Knocks*

"*The Complete Martial Artist* by Willie 'The Bam' Johnson is a fantastic read! Johnson shows through his engaging life story that winning alone does not develop your strengths, your struggles also develop your strengths. His book outlines a solid and practical code of conduct that he recommends to be followed by martial artists. This book goes far beyond just physical martial arts techniques to give you a profound learning experience. Highly recommended for those who want to make martial arts a meaningful way of life!"

—Andrew Zerling, veteran martial artist, multi-award winning author,
Sumo for Mixed Martial Arts: Winning Clinches, Takedowns, and Tactics

"Great Work Mr. Johnson. You are a blessing to many. Keep up your greatness. God Bless."

—Robert L. Wallace, CEO, Birthgroup Technologies, author of
Let God Be God and *Black Wealth: Your Road to Small Business Success*

The Complete Martial Artist

Developing the mind, body, and spirit of a champion

Willie "The Bam" Johnson
Seventh-Degree Black Belt
Seven-Time World Champion

with Nancy Musick
First-Degree Black Belt

 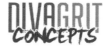

YMAA Publication Center
Wolfeboro, New Hampshire

YMAA Publication Center, Inc.
PO Box 480
Wolfeboro, New Hampshire, 03894
United States of America
1-800-669-8892 • info@ymaa.com • www.ymaa.com

ISBN: 9781594396533 (print) • ISBN: 9781594396540 (ebook)

Copy editor: Doran Hunter
Cover design: Axie Breen
This book typeset in Times LT Std
Illustrations courtesy of the author, unless otherwise noted.

POD 0819

Publisher's Cataloging in Publication

Names: Johnson, Willie, 1964– author. | Musick, Nancy, 1942– author.
Title: The complete martial artist : developing the mind, body, and spirit of a champion / Willie "The Bam"
   Johnson ; with Nancy Musick.
Description: Second edition. | Wolfeboro, New Hampshire : YMAA Publication Center, [2019] | Series:
   True wellness. | Revision of the 2001 edition published by Human Kinetics.
Identifiers: ISBN: 9781594396533 | 9781594396540 (ebook) | LCCN: 2019944296
Subjects: LCSH: Martial arts. | Martial arts—Psychological aspects. | Young adults—Psychology. |
   Self-esteem in young adults. | Young adults—Life skills guides. | Self-actualization (Psychology) | Cognitive
   balance. | Personality development. | Self-realization. | Self-control. | BISAC: SPORTS & RECREATION /
   Martial Arts & Self-Defense. | HEALTH & FITNESS / Exercise / General. | YOUNG ADULT
   NONFICTION / Social Topics / Self-Esteem & Self-Reliance. | YOUNG ADULT NONFICTION /
   Social Topics / Values & Virtues. | YOUNG ADULT NONFICTION / Sports & Recreation / Martial Arts.
Classification: LCC: GV1101 .J64 2019 | DDC: 796.8—dc23

The author and publisher of the material are NOT RESPONSIBLE in any manner whatsoever for any injury that may occur through reading or following the instructions in this manual.

The activities, physical or otherwise, described in this manual may be too strenuous or dangerous for some people, and the reader(s) should consult a physician before engaging in them.

Warning: While self-defense is legal, fighting is illegal. If you don't know the difference, you'll go to jail because you aren't defending yourself. You are fighting—or worse. Readers are encouraged to be aware of all appropriate local and national laws relating to self-defense, reasonable force, and the use of weaponry, and act in accordance with all applicable laws at all times. Understand that while legal definitions and interpretations are generally uniform, there are small—but very important—differences from state to state and even city to city. To stay out of jail, you need to know these differences. Neither the author nor the publisher assumes any responsibility for the use or misuse of information contained in this book.

Nothing in this document constitutes a legal opinion nor should any of its contents be treated as such. While the author believes that everything herein is accurate, any questions regarding specific self-defense situations, legal liability, and/or interpretation of federal, state, or local laws should always be addressed by an attorney at law.

When it comes to martial arts, self-defense, and related topics, no text, no matter how well written, can substitute for professional, hands-on instruction. These materials should be used for academic study only.

Printed in USA.

In loving memory of my mother, Martha Wellons Johnson, who gave me life and showed untiring support and commitment in helping me become a martial artist.

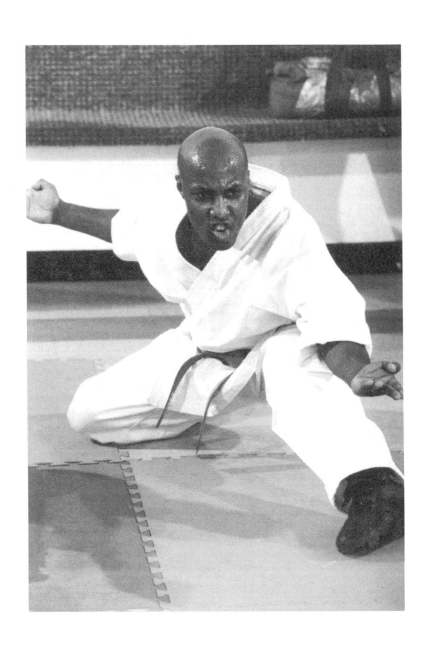

Contents

Preface

When this book was first published nearly twenty years ago, the editor and I agreed that if it weren't for the drills and techniques, the book could be marketed in the self-help/inspiration category. My greatest hope for it was that my story would inspire others to change their lives for the better.

Today, at the suggestion of publisher David Ripianzi, this book is being republished at a time when people seem more lost, and our society more violent, than when I began working on it in my jail cell in 1989. Writing it was my way of cleansing myself, learning to love myself for the first time, and to just plain man up as I struggled to become a complete human being. In the end, there turned out to be no struggle and no real incompleteness; all I had to "do" was to be in the now and manifest the truth that was already inside of me.

As I moved forward in my new life, I tried to demonstrate by my own example that being a complete martial artist is not about money in the bank, rewards, belts, or titles. It's about learning to optimize mind, body, and spirit in order to be a godly man or woman, good father or mother, good husband or wife, successful business-person, or great community leader. A complete martial artist lives fully in the now, always mindful of what the present circumstances are calling him to do.

While I was incarcerated and hopeless, I joined a group called Who Are You. One of the group members, a man everyone knew as Brother D, broke me down so he could build me back up and show me the inner strength I didn't know I had. He taught me that real strength comes from faith and the ability to adapt and flow in harmony with the universe. While I was on that journey of transformation, a light came on from within me, and I began to live and express my true self.

So, as you read this book, remember the journey is now. Being and staying in the moment is all we have; it's our only reality.

At my martial arts academy, our focus is on changing lives everywhere, from the suburbs to the hood. Millions of people have been impacted by the complete martial artist way we teach, and the authentic truth contained within it is needed today more than at any point in my lifetime. As a martial arts teacher, I have found that teaching technique is secondary to nurturing human development, especially of young people. Many children are broken because parents, leaders, and teachers are themselves broken and incomplete. Their egos won't let them see how they are standing in their own way. Patterns of dysfunction get passed on to the children and the cycle continues over and over. In our work in the martial arts, my family and I have set out to disrupt that cycle. What we do is bigger than a martial arts practice. It's about helping others become not only complete martial artists but complete human beings.

There was a time when martial arts played a role in every area of human existence. In all parts of the world, each culture had its unique expression of the martial arts that was based on the cultural and historical circumstances of the people. The driving force behind the structure, techniques, and applications in each martial arts system was the need to defend against an attack and survive. The martial arts were also a way of life.

Today, although there are still situations where the martial arts can save your life, their primary uses are in sports, entertainment, and spiritual transformation. More and more people, however, are discovering how aspects of the traditional martial arts can be applied to today's fast-paced, often frantic lifestyles.

The martial arts are taught under many banners (such as karate, gongfu, jujitsu, taekwondo), but they all revolve around the same basic values and principles. These principles include honesty, persistence, courage, self-expression, and creativity, all of which are meant to promote individual growth and help you create a balanced approach to living. Regardless of which martial art you practice or your level of experience, this book will show you ways to improve your physical performance and help you achieve harmony of body, mind, and spirit for success not only in the martial arts but also in life. Even if you are not a martial artist but an athlete, fitness instructor, or just someone dedicated to being the best you can be, you'll discover important tools to help you develop your individual expression. *The Complete Martial Artist* shows you how to find balance and harmony within yourself and with the universe, which is what everyone strives for in and out of the martial arts.

Chapter 1, "The Pursuit of Do," describes some of the significant events in my life as I pulled myself up from addiction and incarceration to being a seven-time world champion. By sharing what I've learned during my ups and downs, I hope you'll be able to apply the lessons I learned to your own life. You'll discover the drive within yourself to pursue your goals, meet your challenges, and reach beyond your limits. I also teach you how to use your creativity and imagination to reach your goals, face your fears, and use the negative as a stepping stone to the positive. This chapter starts you on a never-ending quest for self-improvement, which is what the pursuit of Do is about.

Chapter 2, "Universal Principles," introduces you to *wushudo*—your road map for developing physical, mental, and spiritual fitness. The twelve universal principles at the heart of wushudo will strengthen your martial arts performance and make your travels through life easier and more satisfying. This chapter helps you attain the highest level of martial arts training. At this level, you have the ability to perform beyond all boundaries, systems, styles, and techniques with total freedom of self-expression. You'll learn the importance of adopting a diverse training philosophy that focuses on fitness, forms, weapons, self-defense, and self-understanding.

Chapter 3, "Champion Attitude," offers you a powerful and effective weapon to add to your arsenal—the mind-set of a champion. You must learn how to use your mind as a tool for reaching your full potential. This chapter shows you how to exercise champion qualities like discipline, concentration, and determination in practice and in competition. By adopting the right attitude, you'll not only improve your martial arts skills but also learn to not let anything stand in the way of reaching your goals.

Chapter 4, "Katas and Weapons," takes what you've learned in previous chapters and applies it to katas and weapons practice. You'll go beyond executing techniques to expressing your true nature. The drills in this chapter will improve your focus, fluidity, balance, endurance, coordination, and confidence. Your techniques will become more reflexive, improving your ability to react quickly and effectively in competition or in a self-defense situation. Furthermore, you'll be able to apply the improved dexterity and confidence you gain from kata practice to your everyday life.

Chapter 5, "Freestyle Sparring," describes how to develop the free mind, responses, and reflexes needed to outthink and outmaneuver your opponent, whether in the ring or on the street. The drills and fighting concepts in this chapter will arm you with the tools you need to be a great freestyle fighter. You'll learn how to bring together all the physical elements and natural fighting techniques with speed and fluidity. This chapter covers the principles of effective sparring, along with tips on kicking, grappling, ground fighting, and hand techniques. Each series of photos shows you the proper way to execute takedowns, sweeps, leads, and counters. In addition, you'll learn important keys to winning, such as taking your time, staying aware of your surroundings, controlling your emotions, and following your instincts.

The last chapter, "The Road to Success," reveals how to start something and see it through to a successful conclusion. Although it's always easy to start something new, the challenge is to stay dedicated. This chapter contains tips to help keep you moving toward your goals. It covers choosing a training facility; building strength, endurance, and flexibility; practicing good nutrition; having the right attitude; and expressing yourself through the martial arts. You'll learn to keep going even when there's no support or rewards—just the satisfaction of knowing you're doing the right thing for the right reasons.

Most books concentrate on either the skills and drills of the martial arts, or on the spiritual aspects. *The Complete Martial Artist* is about developing the whole self physically, mentally, and spiritually. If you understand and apply its principles, you'll be on your way to reaching your goals and realizing your full potential in and out of martial arts. There are no limits to what you can do and who you can become other than the limits you impose on yourself.

Acknowledgements

Special thanks to my mother, Martha Johnson, for always believing in and encouraging me; my father, Willie Johnson, Sr., for teaching me the importance of self-defense; my sister, Celestine (Tiney) Cook; my niece, Miacha Keeling; my children, Marco, Nailah, Shirley, Shamia, Crystal, La Vonda, Marshieh, Zarion, and my step-daughter Joelle; my wife, Kimber; and my spiritual advisors, Mitchell Davis and Nancy Musick.

Thank you to my hero, Bruce Lee; Grand Master Kenneth Parker; Grand Master Tony Lin; Grand Master Garcia Davis; and Mfundi Tayari Casel. A special thank-you to the one person who has always been here for me, in good times and bad, treating me with unconditional love—Grand Master Dennis Brown, my martial arts father.

Thank you to every student I have ever had; every parent who brought a child to me to teach; and every martial artist I have ever trained with, competed against, spoken a word to, or read about. In some way, large or small, you each touched my life and helped me become the person I am today.

Thank you, God, for letting me experience all that I have, both positive and negative. Through these experiences I have searched for and found the man I am today.

Willie "The Bam" Johnson

Thank you to Willie Johnson—my instructor, friend, and soul mate—for allowing me to walk with you on this incredible journey called life; to my parents, Alden and Dorothy Holt, for giving me my foundation; and to my children, Michael, James, and Diane, for their understanding and patience with my dedication to the martial arts.

Thank you to each and every martial artist I have had the pleasure to train with: my seniors who lead the way, my peers who walk with me, and my juniors who allow me to share my newfound knowledge.

Thank you, God, for the gifts You have so freely given me. May I in turn repay them to others ten thousand-fold.

Nancy Musick

Author's Note

I promise...

To be the best I can be and have a wonderful, honest life.

To rely in my faith in the creator and have the willpower to go and Let God. I will seek to set goals that complement the inner me and not ones based on worldly opinions. Most importantly, I will leave the results up to God, no matter what.

This year of 1989, I will stop being blind, open my eyes and stop the insane behavior. I will not lie, steal, use drugs or give up in the midst of struggle. I know if I don't fight those insane behaviors, I will continue to live behind these jail bars.

So I promise God and myself on June 11, 1989, that I will never lose my freedom again. I know that with true freedom comes responsibility and on this day, expressing my freedom responsibly is my quest.

I live this promise still to this day and will for the rest of my life.

—Willie "The Bam" Johnson

Introduction

I do not regret the past, nor do I wish to shut the door on it, because without it, I would not be able to make the right choices today.

By the time I was twenty-five, I had become a world champion martial artist with a reputation as a promising martial arts star in America and on the sport karate circuit. I had graduated from the prestigious Beijing Physical Culture Institute in China and had been a guest on popular television shows. During the time I was making a name for myself in the martial arts, however, I was also developing many negative habits to support a worsening drug and alcohol lifestyle. In 1989, the negative side of this double lifestyle finally caught up with me and, despite a promising martial arts career, I found myself behind bars.

The sound of the prison doors closing behind me reached a place deep inside my gut. It is one thing to spend a few days or weeks in the city jail waiting for a hearing; it is another to face an entire year in prison. During past experiences, I had managed to be rescued by my mom from any long-term consequences. This time it was different. No one was coming. My mom had died of cancer several years earlier and now, homeless, addicted to drugs and alcohol, and trying to support a lifestyle far beyond my financial means, my luck had run out. I was sentenced to one year in a minimum-security facility, but for some reason that I still don't know, I arrived at a maximum-security prison and was locked down with the most hardened criminals. My worst nightmare had come true. I always thought I would rather be dead than incarcerated.

What I would soon realize, however, is that my incarceration was a blessing in disguise. Without that year in jail, I wouldn't have had the time to get to know myself. I made myself a promise that I would never lose my freedom again. I spent the year studying and soul-searching, determined to get back on a positive path.

In prison, I left my cell for two hours every evening to participate in a group called "Who Are You?" When you shared anything about yourself in this group, the group facilitator and other group members told you if you were lying or pretending to yourself. They cut through the smokescreen of pompous, self-righteous, tough-guy attitudes and told you who you really were. In another setting, I suppose it would be much like going into group therapy, but this was what prison life offered. While I was telling people how I wanted to help them change the behaviors that support addictive lifestyles, I also faced my drug and alcohol problem. For the first time in my life, I made a conscious decision to look inside myself, feel the pain, and change those things about myself that I could. There weren't a lot of resources in prison for self-improvement; however, religious leaders made a commitment to bring information about spirituality in the format of daily services and group meetings. I frequented these groups. Many men went because it gave them something to do outside their cells or because it looked good on their records when they went for a parole hearing. I had other motives. First, I wanted to hear the messages each carried about the universal truths of their religions. I believed that the Universal Creator was using martial arts as my window of opportunity. Second, I wanted them to read my notes about the principles and truths I felt were important, to see if they matched those universally accepted. Again, I was reaching out for more education and was not only welcomed in these groups but also recognized as a valued participant and group leader.

Before long, I began to bond with different religious leaders—those of the Nation of Islam, Muslims, Baptists, and other denominations of Christianity, to name a few. I didn't claim to be a Christian or a Muslim. My belief was in the Universal Creator, and I was open to all spiritual growth without the boundaries of a particular religion. Nevertheless, they read my notes and commented on many occasions that, yes, my ideas were exactly what they believed and taught. These principles and truths form the foundation for my martial arts curriculum and are set forth in *The Complete Martial Artist.*

It is only through embracing the concepts and skills in this book that I have been able to regain control of my life. Today, I am a seven-time world champion martial artist and founder of the Universal Martial Arts Concepts Academy, but I continue to set new goals and look for ways to improve myself. It is this constant battle for self-improvement that will enable you to discover your balance—physically, mentally, and spiritually.

The Pursuit of Do

The hills and valleys on the path of life are necessary for you to know how much further you have to go to grow.

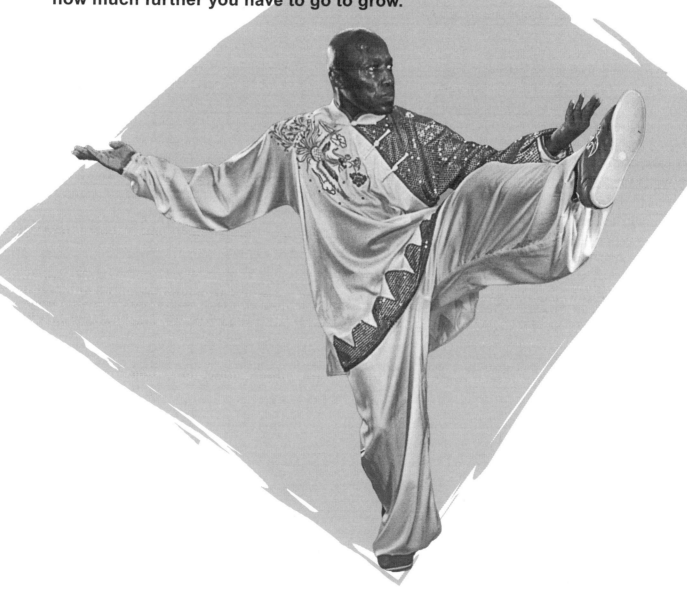

There is a formula in Western civilization that many people follow, hoping for inner peace and happiness—a good education, plus a good job, plus lots of money and material possessions, plus family and friends equal inner peace and happiness. We've all heard this idea before. Yet, when you talk to those who have all this, are they happy? I mean really happy? Probably not. They will say something like, "I have it all, but something's missing. I just don't feel content. I want something else, but I don't know what." They are restless, frequently jumping from one job, hobby, activity, or relationship to another. This is a person who is driven by their unrest in response to external pressures.

On the other hand, have you ever taken the time to seek someone who is happy and content with life? Often the happiest people don't have financial wealth or many material possessions. What is their secret? They have discovered that happiness is an inside job, meaning that you must develop your inner self so you can be happy no matter what life hands you. They are driven from the inside to pursue goals and challenges they have set for themselves. Instead of thinking about what they want to do, they feel what they must do. They have learned to listen to the music of their souls and sing their own songs. Before I got locked up, I felt totally empty. I had spent my life chasing everything I thought would make me happy—new clothes, a new girlfriend, alcohol, drugs. If it meant I had to steal or hurt someone to get what I wanted, I did whatever it took. In jail, I had no idea how to be happy and feel at peace, but for the first time in my life, I had plenty of free time to contemplate. I desperately wanted to feel better about myself than I did at that moment.

While in jail, I began to reflect on my life up to that point and the lessons I had learned. After some time, with help from others around me, I realized that I had to look inside myself to be happy instead of expecting other people, places, and things to bring me happiness. The Japanese call this journey *Do*; the Chinese call it *Dao*. In the proper context, it is a journey that is universal, never ending, and constantly evolving. It recognizes only one enemy, one problem, and that is self. There is a constant battle to improve one's self, a drive to achieve balance, then a conscious effort to maintain that balance. You can only achieve this through simple improvements, constructive changes, and continual progress. When I look at the events of my past, I am now able to recognize which behaviors were destructive and which were beneficial. It is through this type of analysis that I'll avoid reliving my mistakes. Of course, as a child, I simply lived for the moment. It was an exciting time—a time when I first realized my love of martial arts and reveled in the confidence it gave me. My imagination and thirst for knowledge soared. There were times, however, when I let peer pressure take control. Today I realize that each of us holds the answer to any of life's questions—it's inside us. We just have to be open to hearing the message and willing to use it. What follows is an account of some events in my life that eventually lead me on my continual and peaceful journey of Do—one that I will pursue until death. My hope is that by sharing with you what I've learned during this journey, you will be able to take these lessons and apply them to your life and your pursuit of Do.

Follow Your Dreams

It was Bruce Lee's movie *The Chinese Connection* that motivated me to pursue the goal of becoming a martial artist and an action screen hero. I went to see *The Chinese Connection* when I was six years old, and I sat through the movie spellbound. It was love at first sight—love for Bruce Lee, love of the martial arts, and love of movies. I could hardly wait to get home and tell Mom what I had seen.

I'm not sure how many people know from the age of six what they want to do in life, but I did—I wanted to be just like Bruce Lee! I had a burning desire to follow in his footsteps, but my dad thought it was a waste of time. "Be a killer like me," he said, "and forget about being like that Chinese punk." I can't put into words how hurt I felt when he said this. For a minute, I felt like the life was being sucked right out of me, but Mom took me in her arms, comforted me, and told me I could do anything I wanted. She always believed in me, no matter what. My life in Baltimore's inner city didn't come with the advantages that many kids in the suburbs had. There wasn't extra money for anything. Even if there had been a martial arts school in my neighborhood, I couldn't have gone, but I didn't know anything about martial arts

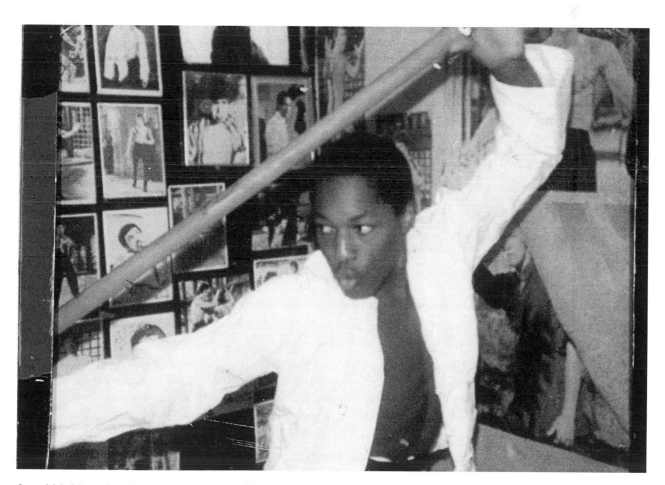

As a kid, I loved to imitate the moves of famous martial artists such as Bruce Lee.

schools. At six years old, you just think you can do whatever you want. So I imitated the moves of the people I saw in movies, books, and magazines, and let my body flow naturally.

Six-year-olds have a wonderful gift of make-believe, and I'm sure I thought I really was Bruce Lee. There was no one to tell me I was doing a technique wrong, and I just adapted what I saw into what my body could do. This natural expression is what our martial arts ancestors displayed before there were structured systems. All true martial arts teachers hope their students won't lose their childlike expression as they travel through today's structured curriculums. It's this expression that gives you flavor.

If there is a dream or a goal you long to accomplish, you should pursue it with all your heart. Go after your dreams with the energy and enthusiasm you knew as a child, and let your curiosity help you push beyond immediate boundaries. In fact, if you are serious about wanting your goals to manifest, write them down, date them, and put them someplace you have to read them every day. For as long as I can remember, every year between Christmas and New Year's Day, I made a list of what I wanted to accomplish in the next year. I even put a date by each goal for when I wanted to achieve it. Then I taped the list to the bathroom mirror so I had to read it every morning and night. More often than not, when the time came, I had reached the goal. One year I didn't make a list, and my life started going downhill in a hurry. I heard a voice telling me to make a list, but I wouldn't listen. The voice also said that if I didn't, I would lose everything. That was in 1989, the year I was incarcerated, so it came true. Today, I wouldn't dream of entering a new year without my goals written down. I review the present strong points and weak points to find a way to continue my strengths and improve my weaknesses. This never-ending quest for self-improvement is what pursuing Do is about.

Surround Yourself with Supportive People

When going after something you love, it's important to surround yourself with people who will encourage and support you. However, if you do encounter people who are trying to influence you in a negative way or tear you down, your focus should always be on what is right for you, regardless of what others tell you.

Living in Baltimore's inner city, we often moved from one housing project to another, so I was always the new kid on the block. This meant I was constantly being picked on and beat up. I remember one bullying encounter I had with my so-called friends. We had been playing football and I had made some good plays. Well, I guess that made one guy mad because he hauled off and hit me several times in the face. When I looked up, figuring that my friends would help me out, they were all walking away, ignoring me. I was scared and wanted this guy to stop hitting me. To make matters worse, he took my shoes, and I had to walk home barefoot.

When I got home, I rushed to my bedroom and shut the door—relieved to be in a safe place. I wondered why I got beat up, and just at the moment when I felt proud and confident about myself. Why would this make someone feel threatened? Today, I know there is a choice. You don't have to be around people who tear you down, or, should I say, you can keep them at a distance. It is important to surround yourself with only those people you can trust to want the best for you. People who really love you won't treat you badly.

> **Surround yourself with only those people you can trust to want the best for you.**

It was my older sister, Celestine (Tiney, for short), who came to my rescue and taught me how to protect myself. Martial arts only put some polish on my fighting—my big sister taught me how to stand up for myself. At home, my dad mentally abused me instead of helping me learn how to protect myself. Everyone was afraid of my dad, including me, so when he called me a punk, a chump, or worse, it destroyed any self-esteem I had.

Today, as a parent and teacher, I try to be compassionate about my children's and students' struggles by listening, using tough love, and giving unconditional support. I feel it is a juggling act when you help others through something. You must feel when to step in or when to back up and let go. If you force a solution, you can break the natural flow and interfere with the outcome. You have to get out of the middle so others can find the solution that is right for them. You always have the answer you need—just look inside.

One unforgettable experience was when I was confronted at a neighborhood crap game by a guy who was a great wrestler and who had taken my money in the past. Everyone was afraid of him, including me. I was standing there shooting craps, and he came up, socked me in the chest, and told me to give him my money. I started kicking and punching him until he put me in a headlock. I got loose and started acting crazy—doing karate moves and screaming as I had seen in the movies. On the inside I was scared to death, but I was tired of being bullied. Believe it or not, this guy let me go and never bothered me again. This seemed to be a turning point, because others started to respect and fear me. Today I teach my kids and students to keep themselves out of negative situations and away from negative people if possible. If you can't, though, you have to be ready to stand up and fight. In the old days, adults in the housing projects made us fight it out, and afterward we were friends. Today, these encounters end in death by guns or knives, so it is important to be aware of your choices if you encounter a bully.

Life is full of challenges, and as I've gotten older, the challenges have moved away from physical confrontations to emotional and mental hurdles—someone is always trying to make you lose focus on what's right for you. This kind of person is like a snake creeping up on you and attacking you from nowhere when you least expect it. So no matter what someone tries to do to you, no one has the power to make you feel bad unless you allow it.

During your journey you will come across people who want to hurt you or see you fail. Their negative influence will hinder your quest only if you let it. Take care to surround yourself with people who are trustworthy, reliable, and respectful.

Resist External Pressures

Although you should associate with people who will be a positive influence on you, the same goes for the way you treat others. If you fail to listen to yourself—to what you know is right or wrong—and let peer pressure take over, you're letting external pressures run your life. Your journey is not your own.

One weekend on my way to the movies, I took my bicycle over to a cousin's house for repairs. While I was there, my aunt sent us to the store for some groceries. I wanted to impress everyone, so I stole some candy and gave it to my cousins. I let peer pressure take control of my actions and did something I knew was wrong. At the time, it was a cool thing to do, and for an instant I felt like a hero on center stage. This wasn't the first time I had stolen something, though. I had been taking small amounts of money from my mom to buy karate magazines, books, posters, and training equipment.

For as long as I can remember, I have been able to attract people to me who want to do whatever I'm doing—something like a magnetic personality. Then when their backs were turned, I stole from them. Bookstore owners were a favorite of mine. I would go into the store and start a conversation, then walk out with a couple books or magazines under my coat. I used to go to the same stores and sometimes I got caught, but the owners always forgave me with the admonition, "You're a good kid; just don't do it again." But of course, I always did.

One instructor told me I had charisma. People feel confident around me and trust me. Now I use this gift to help people make positive changes in their lives and to be a good role model for them, but when I was selling drugs, people followed me down that path, too.

On the streets, if you want respect, you and your homeboys have to do crazy things. Because my specialty was stealing, I would go into stores and steal for our gang, which got its name from a martial arts movie called *Seven Blows of the Dragon*. In the movie, there was a gang of bandits called "Mountain Brothers" who stole from the rich and gave to the poor. We were so impressed by these movie bandits that we named ourselves after them and made weapons like they used. I carried two small sticks on my back and a long stick in my hands. Finally, I didn't feel like the little kid who everyone bullied. I had earned the respect of the neighborhood cool guys, and there was no turning back. They had become my extended family, and I would do anything for them.

As all gangs, we did bad things like breaking into the bakery and warehouses, and so on. Several times we were caught, but my mom was always there to rescue me. Back then, the police just kept you in a room and talked to you until your parents showed up to take you home. I never saw the inside of a jail cell until much later. My dad always sat me down and talked to me about staying out of trouble and not going to jail like he had. I listened, but when the peer pressure came, I got swept away and went right back to doing bad things.

Encountering a Bully

When you come across a bully, it is important to understand that there are several defensive tools you can use to escape a fight. To avoid these situations altogether, it helps to know what types of bullies there are and what weapons they will use to try to put you down.

Principles of Bullies

- Verbal bullies know how to say things that hurt you at just the time your guard is down or when you are in the presence of others.
- Practical joker bullies have the ability to crack jokes on you or play games that put you down in front of others and make you feel ridiculous.
- Athletic bullies use physical prowess to abuse you, hoping they will embarrass and hurt you.
- Authoritative bullies are in positions of power and use this position to create a double standard, putting themselves outside the rules.
- Intellectual bullies have learned to express their gifted mental talents and abuse you with them to feel superior.
- Spiritual bullies use the words of the Universal Creator to beat you down, trying to prove that they are right and you are wrong. They have no concern for your feelings.
- Chemically dependent bullies are involved with drugs and alcohol and do everything in their power to make you feel less than them because you choose not to use drugs and alcohol.
- Sexual bullies make you feel uncomfortable for not having sex or try to persuade you to have unsafe sex.
- Patriotic bullies try to force their political beliefs on you.
- Financial bullies try to make you feel less than them because they have more money and believe no one without money is of use to them.
- Whining bullies try to make you feel sorry for them so they can get what they want.
- Prejudiced bullies put you down because they feel as though their race, religion, or way is superior to all others, and they will go to any lengths to prove this.

Defensive Tools

- Conduct yourself in a positive manner, being careful that you don't respond to bullies negatively. Treat them as you would like to be treated.
- Be humble, making sure you aren't a show-off when you make new friends. Take charge of your behavior by working the first two defensive tools.
- Never underestimate anyone, because sometimes the quiet or weak-appearing person is the most dangerous.
- Try to be friends with bullies by using humor in a nonthreatening way. Walk away from bullies and talk to someone in authority the first time you feel insulted.

- Never give bullies a chance to treat you the same way twice.
- Hang out with people who strive to be of good character like you and make no exceptions.
- When feeling threatened, use trickery or be in agreement with bullies to resolve the conflict.
- Do your best to prevent conflict by working the previous steps. Even yell, scream, or become tough by acting like the experience had no effect on you. You can reason with bullies, trying to teach them in a nonthreatening way why their behavior is wrong.
- If all else fails, stand and fight to protect yourself and control the situation.

Remember, today the youngest kid has weapons, and some will come back for revenge after someone stands up to them. So be careful and do your very best to prevent fighting.

Show Respect for Others

In the projects, this was a time when everyone was close. They looked out for each other and for each other's kids. This was a good time to be growing up—we just played differently. The values and character traits that I have today came from this family village upbringing. They lived the saying, "It takes a whole village to raise a child."

Things mellowed out between the gangs, and I got interested in playing baseball, basketball, and football in my neighborhood. I joined a Little League baseball team put together by a community not far from ours called Little Italy. These Italian Americans were reaching out to the African American community, hoping that we could come together in a spirit of peace and harmony.

Neighborhood store owners gave us free soft drinks and candy, and the coaches had cookouts for us and invited us to their homes to watch the major leagues play on television. During these times of fun and excitement, no one ever thought that someday these fun-loving kids would get into the deadly game of drugs.

In my family, my parents taught me the right way to treat adults and gave me a foundation of principles. I think what my parents taught me gave me an edge over other gang members. I talk with many people today who honestly believe that if you grew up in the projects, you had to come from a bad home. That just isn't true. My mom and dad worked hard to provide for us. They always found a way for us to have good holidays and the necessities of everyday life. I never went without food or clothes or, most importantly, love. We were a family that did everything together—even sitting down together at mealtime!

This is the way I was taught to show respect for others, and I teach the same principles to my students. Most people think I learned good manners from studying martial arts, but that only complemented what I was learning at home. My dad, regardless of his personal choices in life, was a great teacher for me in every aspect of my life. He is the toughest, yet the most honest, man I have ever been around. If he doesn't like you, he lets you know it. At the same time, he would do anything to protect his family, even if it meant dying.

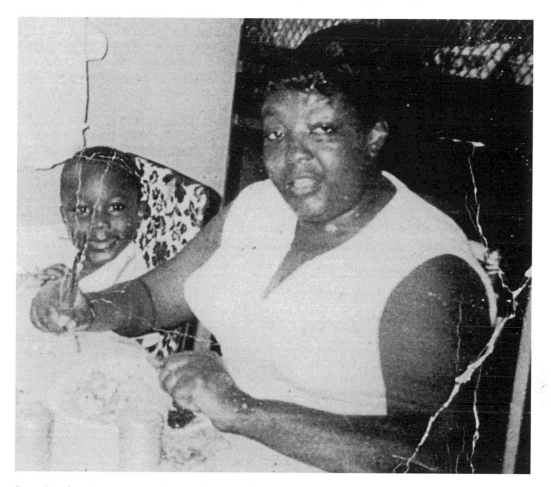

Despite the struggles we faced living in the inner city, my mom made sure we never went without love.

You'll never reach a sense of peace and balance in your life if you do not show respect for others. Display trust and love to others to make a positive influence on their lives. Practice being part of the solution; otherwise you're part of the problem.

> Practice being part of the solution;
> otherwise you're part of the problem.

Use Your Creativity and Imagination

Regardless of the circumstances, with a little creativity and a lot of determination, you can accomplish anything. In fact, there are no limits to what you can achieve, only those you place on yourself.

Funding for Little League baseball stopped. The kids who had been taken out of the projects into a better community, one where we were united with people of all races, were back on the streets with nothing to do. Creativity kicked in, as it always does, and we began to compete with a new sport called street gymnastics. We learned this by taking old, filthy mattresses and box springs, setting them on top of each other, then practicing flips. My confidence soared, and suddenly I had heart to flip on concrete, and off rooftops, cars, fences, walls, and everything I came across. I got so interested in gymnastics that it was natural to combine it with my martial arts. I had found something to get the attention of other martial artists, and it gave me an edge.

By the time I was eleven, Tiney had moved into a place of her own, and I took advantage of her empty bedroom, turning it into a home gym. I had Bruce Lee posters all over the walls and every type of homemade training equipment you can imagine—wing chun wooden dummies, sandbags, speed bags, and several martial arts weapons. I also had an extensive library of fighting books. I spent my days training and immersing myself in martial arts. It never occurred to me that I couldn't succeed in martial arts because I didn't have the best equipment or a school to train in. I did sit-ups, push-ups, jumping jacks; went running; practiced forms and shadowboxing—anything I could think of to keep me moving toward my goal to be like Bruce Lee. Few people can have all the right equipment or a perfect training environment. It's the ones who are willing to make do with what they have and go forward who are the hard-core, self-made martial artists like our ancestors.

> Few people have all the right equipment or a perfect training environment. It's the ones who are willing to make do with what they have and go forward who are the hard-core, self-made martial artists like our ancestors.

Use Your Mind

While I was physically training, reading began to play an important part in my life. Because I was curious about everything, I went into bookstores and stayed for hours reading books about martial arts, boxing, wrestling, gymnastics, and everything that grabbed my attention.

I learned that books paint pictures of dreams in words the same way movies do, but with one difference. When you read something, it gets inside your head and makes you think. It triggered my imagination at a deep level, and I was soon reading philosophy books about Confucianism, Daoism, Buddhism, the yin and yang concept, and technical books by Bruce Lee, S. Henry Cho, and Master Oyama, to name a few. Of course, I didn't understand a lot of what I was reading, but the words seemed to soothe a place deep inside me, so I read as best I could.

It wasn't until I was in jail that I began to understand these things. I was reading similar books, only now I was old enough to feel and understand what they were saying. It felt like I was revisiting things of the past and remembering. I had come to realize that others were respecting me for this talent when, one day, when I was going out to the yard, an inmate I had never spoken with came up to me and gave me a book on Eastern philosophy. I began to read it and cross-reference it with my notes on my martial arts curriculum, and they were connected. I took this as a sign of approval for me from the Universal Creator.

When parents come to my school and complain that our students' creed and some of the rules are beyond what their kids can understand, I smile and tell them, "It's OK; it will be good discipline for them, and they will grow to understand the rules." I do this because I know from my experience it will happen.

Don't Take No for an Answer

My determination and eagerness to learn were paying off, and I was making a name for myself throughout the neighborhood. More and more kids wanted me to teach them martial arts. However, my home gym was overflowing with homemade equipment, so it was time to look for a larger training space. McKim's Community Center was across the street, so, only a preteen, I marched in and asked to speak to the manager, who asked for my credentials to teach martial arts. I was shocked! No one had ever asked me for documents saying I should be allowed to teach martial arts. Of course, the manager told me no.

Instead of stopping me, it added fuel to my burning desire to teach. I started walking to every martial arts school I could get to, talking with the instructors, watching classes, picking up tips on techniques, and so on. I walked miles to get to these schools.

Finally, I found a boxing gym that let me train for free and someone who gave me kick boxing lessons. Still, my students and I were practicing street gymnastics for hours each day, along with the martial arts curriculum I had written, and usually in full view of the community center's manager.

Before long, we were invited in by a counselor named Kenneth Parker. We gave Mr. Parker a demonstration of what we could do and begged him to start a martial arts club for us. Wonder of wonders, that's exactly what Mr. Parker did. Mr. Parker was a martial artist in his own right, teaching kang duk kwan, wing chun, judo, yoga, and gymnastics. This was the first time I had met a martial arts teacher who was interested in helping me learn.

Our relationship blossomed as we worked hand in hand to achieve success. We watched all the martial arts movies and collected every book on martial arts. He often said I was like Bruce Lee, far ahead of my time, and that my enthusiasm for the arts motivated him to grow mentally and spiritually. I was his prize student, and he let everyone know it.

I always had the drive to stand out from the crowd and be unique, and now Mr. Parker was supporting me and believing in me. Aside from this, Mr. Parker was a certified yoga instructor, and he taught me this meditation art. Without knowing it, I began to get spiritually fit and reconnected to the Universal Creator of my childhood. This was one of the biggest blessings I've ever received. In 1976, Master Kenneth Parker awarded me my first black belt.

I learned that a true test of your drive and endurance is hearing the word no. You can either accept this answer and give up, or, if your goal means something to you, persist until you find a way to make it happen. With hard work and faith, you can find a way to achieve your goals.

> A true test of your drive and endurance is hearing the word no. You can either accept this answer and give up or persist until you find a way to achieve your goals.

Another test of my commitment came when I started writing letters to movie companies in Hong Kong and Japan. Their usual reply was, "Get magazine coverage and win lots of tournament championships—then the movies will come to you." Once, I got a letter back from a magazine saying I was crazy and needed to see a psychiatrist. I was shocked. All I had done was express my feelings about what I wanted in life, and for this they were telling me I was a nut case. To make matters worse, Mom brought the letter up every chance she got, which hurt my feelings, but I didn't quit. If anything, I became motivated to work harder at what I believed was right for me.

Your dreams are *your* dreams, and you can't get upset when someone else doesn't believe in them or support you. You're the only one who can see and feel your dreams. It's a waste of time to try to convince someone else to follow your dreams because they're busy with their own dreams.

Never Underestimate Your Opponent

While I was studying martial arts, I was also doing serious gymnastics training for the Junior Olympics. I placed second on the trampoline and seventh on the floor exercise. The medals I won made me a hero in my school and neighborhood. This was my first taste of getting an award, and I liked it. In fact, I loved it and wanted more, more, more. Tiney and I went to a martial arts tournament so I could see everything the competitors did—the forms, the weapons, the fighting—then I went home and practiced.

After all my practice, I got my first chance to compete in a tournament and test my sparring skills at the Baltimore Karate Championships. When they called me into the ring, I saw that my opponent had no legs. I said, "No, I can't fight him!" On the streets, that would have been a violation of the unspoken code. I also remember thinking, "This guy is handicapped so he's no challenge for me—I will smoke him." The referee said, "Are you just going to quit?" Well, I couldn't do that either, so I fought, and it was a mighty tough fight.

My opponent was already on the floor so I had to go there to meet him. I used a combination of ground fighting techniques, such as monkey boxing, wrestling, ground boxing, tumbling, and street fighting. We tied up before I finally beat him.

Remember that old expression your grandmother used to tell you, "Don't judge a book by its cover"? Well, by the end of the match I had a lot of respect for my opponent.

Most people think I made up this story, but it's true. Until that moment, I didn't realize my training had prepared me to fight from all ranges of combat and as it happens on the street. I learned that you can train in boxing or martial arts classes to learn fighting techniques, but in the real world you have to adjust to the situation no matter what it is. I train to meet my opponents at their level, then execute my style and techniques victoriously. I learned you should never underestimate your opponent.

Condition Your Body

Winning that match put me in place to fight one of Baltimore's toughest fighters, Avon Thomas. This fight had me standing on my feet, but even so, we tied and went into overtime. Then I took a shot to the body and lost, three to two. This was the first time someone hit me in the gut so hard that it took the fight right out of me. Afterward, I went to the gym and did some serious training to tighten up my weaknesses so it would never happen again.

From this I learned a valuable lesson: always condition your body because techniques alone aren't enough. As the saying goes, if you're going to dish it out, you'd better be able to take it. So I work myself and my students like no one else would ever work us. Then, if they experience something like I did in that match, I hope they will be able to suck it up—meaning move, breathe, and relax to make pain their friend. If you can master this, then when opponents hit you with their best shots, it won't bother you. That will destroy your opponents' plans, and you'll love it. Just ask any real fighter.

> Always keep your body in good condition,
> because fatigue will make cowards of us all.

Message from Mr. Parker

One of the most pioneering and innovative martial artists I've ever met or trained with is Shifu Willie "The Bam" Johnson. From the time I first met him when he was about thirteen years old, he had the desire to be one of the best karate warriors ever.

Bam Bam, as we used to call him, would sit attentively at my kriya yoga classes absorbing all a young man's mind and body could. What amazed me was that at the end of our sessions, he and several of his peers would start flipping and tumbling off the walls, steps, and mats at McKim's Community Center where I was teaching and working at the time. One day Bam approached me and said respectfully, "Mr. Parker, I heard you know about karate." I humbly told him yes. It was this young, ambitious boy, Willie "The Bam" Johnson, who talked me into teaching and starting a karate school at McKim's Community Center in Baltimore, Maryland. He also was the one who turned me on to fulfill my dreams by studying at the Tien Shen Pia Kung Fu School headed by Willie and Tony Lin.

By the time Bam was fifteen, he had seen many martial arts movies, but it was Bruce Lee who influenced him to develop himself into the all-around martial artist he is today. Even then, Bam was ahead of his time, because in his small room in the low-rise projects, he had pictures, weapons, and equipment (most of which he made himself). To see a young man, age fifteen, with so much insight was amazing.

As the years passed, Bam came to me with ideas about plays, movie scripts, and books that he would write. He also started studying hard in school, began taking acting and drama classes, and trained with top black belt instructors in the area, such as Master Garcia Davis and many others. Of all the athletes, it was Bam who won competition after competition.

We meditated (Agnihotra, Yajnya), did karate, boxing, wrestling, and so on, and did several fund-raising demonstrations for McKim's Community Center. Willie "The Bam" Johnson always stood out with his performances, giving his best, second to none.

Even though I run my own martial arts academy today, self and God supporting, I still consider the young Master Willie "The Bam" Johnson, born in 1964—the Year of the Dragon—to be one of my top instructors, friends, students, and adopted brothers. Bam is a natural talent, and in my book he is "the Last Dragon."

Sincerely,
Sijo/Shifu Kenneth C. Parker

Face Your Fears

There are bound to be times when fear and anxiety threaten to keep you from pursuing your goals. If you take a chance and have faith, you can overcome the challenges that stand in your way.

At the Baltimore Karate Championships, I'd taken my martial arts to a new level and my self-confidence soared. Following the careers of such martial arts superstars as Cynthia Rothrock, Billy Blanks, Dennis Brown, George Chung, Chuck Norris, and Bill Wallace suddenly became important. It was time to work on a serious plan of attack for winning, so that when my opportunity came I would be prepared.

The big moment arrived at Henry Cho's All American Open at New York's Madison Square Garden—one of the biggest tournaments on the East Coast. The good news was that I had trained hard to meet the challenge. The bad news was that I had a gigantic fear of New York City because of stories I'd heard all my life about the gangs, killers, prostitutes, and so on. Also, I was going alone! Now this was a challenge I wasn't prepared for.

Then something wonderful happened. A counselor at the community center helped me get myself together for the four-hour bus trip to the Big Apple. It was a growing-up stage for me—a 16-year-old kid getting on a bus to New York by himself. On the trip, I kept thinking, when it's time to follow through with something, the only one there to walk with you is the Universal Creator.

Once I got to Madison Square Garden, my anxiety was replaced with confidence and determination. All those long hours of training would put me up on center stage in the evening's Grand Championships—I just knew it. In the daytime, I competed in katas and fighting, taking fourth place in each. Then the blessing came. I tied with one of New York's best weapons people and won the tiebreaker. It was great. Everyone came to me talking about how great my weapons kata was.

I made it to the Grand Championships, as I knew I would. My competition would be with a movie star and a master martial artist. I was ecstatic. Then life kicked in, and I remembered my bus left early and I had no money for a hotel. I had to make a choice. Getting safely back to Baltimore won out, but I was so happy about the win (and relieved to be leaving the city) that it felt like the right thing to do. The lesson I learned that night is when you take chances, have faith and leave the outcome in the Universal Creator's hands, He will protect you. You must have faith, even if that means you don't get what you want that minute. I knew my time would come; now it was time to go home.

Use Your Ingenuity

As luck would have it, another person surfaced who would teach me martial arts, Master Garcia Davis. He took me and a group of his black belts to the top martial arts events on the East Coast. My horizons were broadening.

For the first time, I felt like a martial arts champion. I was making a name for myself on the tournament circuit and I loved competing. Then reality hit me—to be nationally ranked, you have to compete in tournaments all over the country, but how was I going to get there by myself with no money?

I learned that it takes a little ingenuity to think of ways to reach your goals. My strategy was to write letters and send photos to different companies with the hope that someone would sponsor me in tournaments or help me break into films. It worked. The 7-Eleven chain of convenience stores agreed to contribute money, as did Mr. Broadway Payne, owner of a McDonald's restaurant in Baltimore, and McKim's Community Center.

Soon I became a two-time All-American Champion, and I thought the world was mine. Magazines were writing about me and local television shows were offering me interviews. I was honored as one of Baltimore's best, along with Oprah Winfrey, at the Lyric Opera House in Baltimore by Governor William Donald Schaffer. *Karate Illustrated* magazine, now called *Karate-Kung Fu Illustrated,* recognized me as one of America's best national competitors.

Then, one day I read an advertisement in a magazine for Master Dennis Brown's Shaolin Wu-Shu Academy. Master Brown was one of my heroes. He was at all the tournaments, in all the magazines, and had even made a movie or two. The ad gave a telephone number. I took a chance, dialed the number, and Master Brown answered. Chills ran through my body, and I was at a loss for words. This was a major turning point in my life.

Soon thereafter, Master Brown watched me perform at the Red Shields Tournament, where I placed second in forms, weapons, and fighting. I gave him a gymnastics

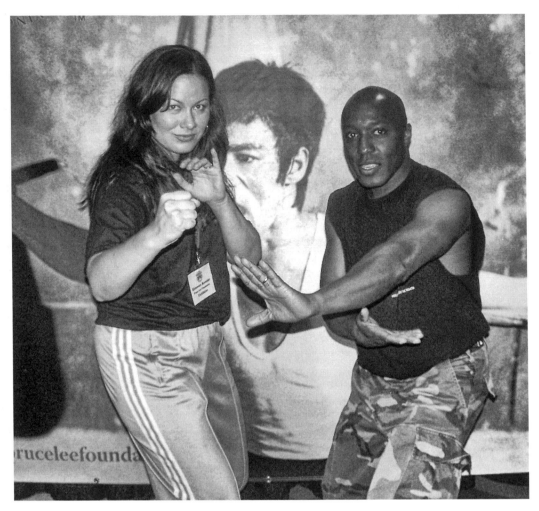

The author with Shannon Lee.

demonstration, which I hoped looked as if I had professional training instead of flipping on mattresses and climbing up brick walls. He must have liked what he saw, because from that day on, Master Brown drove to Baltimore, picked me up, took me to his school in Washington, DC, to practice, and taught me himself. I remember my first time riding with him; it was like a dream. I was so nervous that all I could say was how great he was. His words to me were, "My little brother, I am not great. As a matter of fact, you can achieve the same things I have if you really want them and display good character." I was thrilled beyond words.

What's more amazing is that throughout all this, my former teacher, Mr. Parker, was excited for me. He never shielded me from growing or tried to control me like most instructors do. Today, I follow his example by encouraging my students to identify their strengths, set goals that feel right for them, and follow through.

Identify your strengths and weaknesses,
set goals that feel right for you, and follow through.

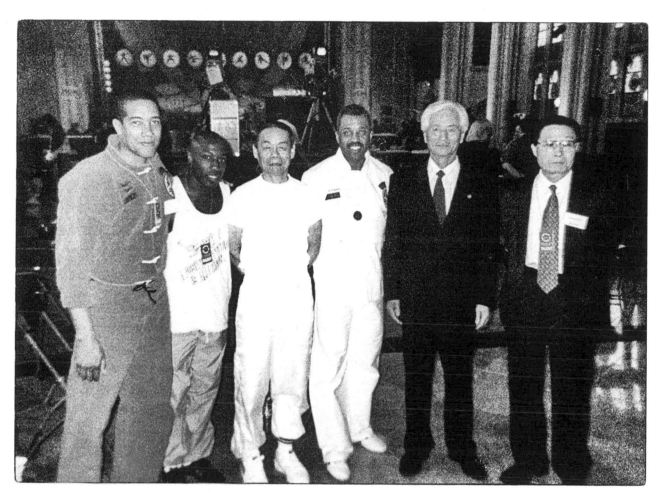

From Left to Right: Grand Master Jhun Rhee, Willie "The BAM" Johnson, Grand Master Bong So Hon, Master Dennis Brown, S. Henry Cho and Master Ervin Master Dennis Brown opened me up to new worlds both in and out of the martial arts.

Withstand the Negative Pull

In the midst of this good fortune, I was aware of the world outside martial arts. Back in my neighborhood, guys were making thousands of dollars a minute selling drugs and walking around with lots of money in their pockets. Drug trafficking was bigger than ever, and with that went plenty of killing and other crime.

Change of Environment

Master Brown asked me if I'd like to live at his school for the summer and do some intense training. It sounded good to me, and I said yes. I had been looking for a way to change my environment, because my homeboys were pressuring me to forget about tournaments and martial arts, saying it was a waste of time. "Heroin is the way to make big money—come and be one of us," they said.

Master Brown brought instructors in to train us for weeks at a time; Cynthia Rothrock, George Chung, Nasty Anderson, Roger Tung, and Tayari Casel, to name a few. For the first time, I had a chance to work out and perform with the best martial artists in the world. I remember them saying I was the competitor they would have to watch out for. This made me work all the harder.

That summer I made the right choice. I followed my heart instead of the lure of drugs and money. If you ever come across this circumstance, make the right choice and look for a way to get out of a bad environment. If you don't, the negative influences may catch up with you, as they did with me.

Turning Point

Dealing drugs was a big lure, and my outgoing personality helped me get girls and get over on people. It was becoming a habit to go out to clubs when I got home from tournaments and celebrate my wins with the guys I used to play basketball with—my homeboys. They bought me things and gave me money and told me I belonged with them. After a few drinks, I believed them.

I remember one time returning home from Orlando, Florida, where I had just won the United States Open Karate Championships. Dad and I were on the way to the store when a friend, who was like a brother to me, stopped us and asked me where I'd been. When I told him of my recent win, he said, "Why not stop by my place and celebrate?" Well, you didn't have to ask me twice to party, but upon entering his house, I saw him shooting drugs and I ran out in disgust.

Because McKim's had given me a key, I headed over there to work out. I must have been there from about 6 to 10 p.m. when I heard gunshots ring out. I was finished at McKim's, so I headed out. On my way home, I saw police and ambulances. I saw someone I knew and asked him what happened. He told me that the friend I caught shooting drugs was killed by another friend over drugs. I was devastated.

I went home, told my parents, and cried myself to sleep. These were the guys I grew up with, played sports with, practiced karate with, went to school with, and now they were killing each other. They were my brothers. The next day, two of the guys involved in the drug war stopped by my house and asked me to take a walk with them. They said that since I had been traveling, all the fun was gone. They wanted me to come back and work with them, like in the old days, and they wanted me to give them an answer that day.

On my way home, all I could think about was my dead friend, the money, and what I could do to get my mom out of the projects. By this time my parents were separated, my dad was busy with his alcoholic friends and had no time for the family, and my mom's health was worsening. She was desperately trying to make ends meet and I was frustrated at not being able to fix the situation. Drug dealing was the big time, and I could be making big money. I needed someone to talk it over with, so I went to my dad. Secretly, I was hoping he would tell me not to get involved, but instead he said, "Do it and get paid." I did just that. My life never was the same again. After that night, I had my own gun and had to report the next day just like I was going to any other job.

If you ever have to make a choice like this, look inside yourself for the answer. Do what you know is right. At the time, I ignored my gut because I thought the positives of drug dealing would outweigh the negatives. Now I know this couldn't be further from the truth. In fact, there are no positives when it comes to that lifestyle.

Negative Effects of Drugs and Alcohol

There were many things I did during this time that I would never have done had I been clean. Instead of being able to hear my voice and listen to what my heart was telling me, I was letting drugs and alcohol control my actions. No matter what you tell yourself, drugs will run your life if you let them.

Our business was in the same fourteen-floor project building I lived in, and we paid the security guard to watch out for us. It was my job to hand the customer the product and take the money. There were two of us who did this, and I couldn't believe the money being made—thousands of dollars in minutes. People came from all over Baltimore to buy drugs from us, and we were so young. The guy in charge was about fifteen.

Eventually, someone put out a hit on my boss. Somehow we all knew about it ahead of time, and the plan was to have the hit man go upstairs, where we would do what was needed. I dreaded encounters like this, because I never wanted anyone to get hurt, but I was so drugged up each day, I didn't think twice about anything any more. The man never came up the stairs, but I was so paranoid—we all were—that the next day I became violent, just like my dad, and insisted we search everyone who entered the building for any reason. Any resistance met with a beating.

A few days later the boss decided to pay the guy back for sending a hit man to get him. So he bought a fish, shot it full of bullet holes, and attached a letter to it that said, "Back off or it's war." Then we paid someone to drop the fish off on the porch of the gang that ordered the hit. These shootouts were commonplace. Life and death meant nothing. It was just the way we lived. Honestly, though, if I hadn't been intoxicated, I never could have done these things.

The money I got in this business was good, more than I've ever seen from any other job I've had. I thought my mom was happy for me and especially for the money I was giving her. Years later, Tiney told me that she was afraid and frightened of me. She didn't know what I'd do and was scared I would get killed. At the time, I was just a kid sitting on what I thought was the top of the world. No adults were stepping up to the plate trying to show us any other way to live. Instead, they were in line buying drugs, asking for money, and stroking our egos.

The Right Choice

For a while, I was able to balance two different lifestyles. I was a successful martial artist who was also dealing drugs, but eventually I had to make a choice. Master Brown hadn't heard from me for almost two months and knew something was wrong. He cared enough about me to drive to my house in the projects and ask my dad to go and get me. When I saw Master Brown, I was embarrassed, even though

I thought he had no idea what I'd been doing. He presented me with the Teacher of the Year Award and the regional forms and weapons titles, and for a moment I felt proud. Before Master Brown left, he said he wanted to meet with me the next week. I had the feeling that my life was going to change, but I didn't know how.

A couple days later, I met with the owner of the local McDonald's, the one who had been sponsoring me in tournament competitions. He said McDonald's wanted to stop my sponsorship and rent me a building for a low monthly price so I could open my own martial arts school. At first I was disappointed, but after I'd had some time to think, I realized they were offering me everything I needed to get out of the drug lifestyle and go straight. I was seventeen at the time and told him I'd get back to him.

When I met with Master Brown, he asked me how I'd like to run a school in Baltimore for him. I shared with him what McDonald's was offering and told him that I had plenty of drug money. We decided to rent the building McDonald's was offering, open a school under Dennis Brown's name, and not use any of my money. I later realized Master Brown knew all along what I was doing and was trying to save me.

Finally, my drug-dealing boss called me in for his own meeting. He thought it was time for me to choose between selling drugs and martial arts—one or the other. I knew in my heart that I wanted to get out of the drug business and find my way back to martial arts and following my goals. I had known for a while that I had become the kid my dad always wanted me to be, and I hated myself. Unless I was high, I couldn't face myself in the mirror or live with my feelings—it just wasn't me. I dug deep to get the courage I needed to walk away, and I headed for the door.

A few days later I heard on the news that my drug-dealing boss was accused of murder, along with a few other people. Looking back over this series of events, I realized that the Universal Creator is always in charge, and all I have to do is listen to the message.

> If you can't face yourself in the mirror,
> it's time to make a change.

Strive for Perfection

Getting out of the drug-dealing business put me back on the right track, and I was more eager than ever to advance my skill level. Following the advice of top martial artists showcased in magazines in the 1980s, I developed a plan of attack for the silver screen. First, I pursued certification as a black belt under qualified martial artists, such as Tony Lin, Garcia Davis, Kenneth Parker, Peter Morales, Dennis Brown, and the Beijing Physical Culture Institute in mainland China. At the same time, I entered the field of sport karate and won numerous national events and a world championship. I was pushing to be the first triple-crown Afro-American martial artist on the circuit. With Master Brown's encouragement, I opened my first school in Baltimore at the ripe old age of seventeen.

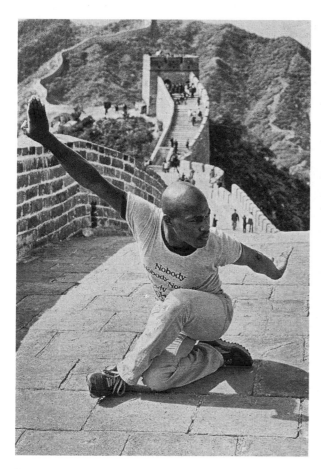

During my trip with Master Brown to the Shaolin Temple School, I trained with some of the best martial artists in the world.

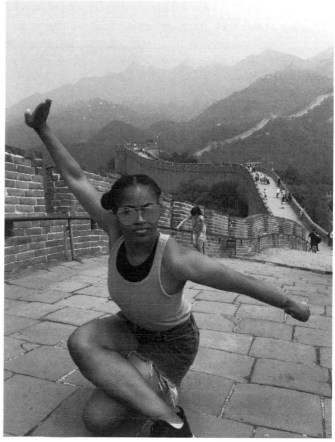

My daughter Nailah recently trained in China, following in my footsteps.

Refine Your Skills

Shortly thereafter, I traveled with Master Brown and a group of his students to mainland China. The purpose of the trip was to help us refine our skills as martial artists, and I hoped to be able to defeat the world's best martial artists. The trip was a great experience. In one month, we saw more than many tourists see in a year. However, the highlight of our trip was to visit, work out, and compete at the Shaolin Temple School. The top coach, head of the Chinese Wu Shu Federation, wanted us to demonstrate our techniques to determine what we knew, what we needed to learn, and how we should be split up. When it came my turn to perform, I gave it my all—jumping, flipping, and twisting with every ounce of warrior spirit I could muster. When I was finished, I saw all the coaches and athletes smiling and talking.

Using our tour guide as the interpreter, they said I was a Shaolinizer, meaning black Shaolin monk. The guide said I was being given this name because my skill level was one of the best they had seen from an American; our team was better than any visiting group that had come there to train. I was ecstatic and trying to be humble at the same time as I walked over to share this moment with Master Brown.

Just then a young man, who I later learned was the full-contact champion of China, tapped me on the shoulder. Our interpreter told me that he wanted to spar with me because he could see I knew how to fight based on the power and spirit exhibited in my form. I asked Master Brown what he thought, and he and the other coaches said OK. He came at me immediately with a whopping leg kick, which told me he was for real. Instinctively I responded with a powerful flurry of punches and kicks, ranging from standing up to the ground. I used my rhythmical footwork to avoid his attack. When the match was over, he asked me if I would train him to fight in exchange for him teaching me wushu techniques. I remember telling him that if Master Brown and my other coaches said it was all right, it was fine with me. Now I had an edge to learning authentic wushu.

That trip reinforced the importance of watching and learning from others. Recognizing the strengths and weaknesses in others, then applying that knowledge to your practice is an excellent way to refine your skills. I went to China eager to learn from the best martial artists in the world. The fact that I was also able to give something back was a thrill beyond words.

Push Yourself

There's no way you can keep getting better if you don't push yourself. The constant quest for self-improvement involves working beyond your current comfort level and not giving up.

Our daily schedule at the Beijing Physical Culture Institute went like this:

From 5:30 to 7 a.m., we prepared for our first two-hour workout, which ran from 7 to 9 a.m. Our next workout was from 12 noon to 2 p.m., and the third was from 4 to 6 p.m. This was instructor-led training. Between these sessions, we practiced on our own and as a team. I knew I had to hang in there and not give up for anything. I held every stance to the lowest level and did every kick slowly and precisely to develop extraordinary control. After the next couple workouts, I was leading my group, pushing everyone to their highest level, and encouraging them not to hold anything back.

> Self-improvement comes only when you push yourself
> beyond your current comfort level.

Adopt Martial Arts as a Way of Life

When I began my trip to China, I was focused on only what I would gain physically—improvement in my forms and weapons. After living side by side with my Chinese wushu brothers and sisters for a month, observing the ways of the Chinese people, I realized something else. The people didn't just practice wushu, the physical aspect of the martial art. They embraced it mentally and spiritually as part of their lives, from the youngest to the oldest, in the city or the country. I was amazed and still am. It was a turning point for me, and at that moment I decided I wanted to live wushu, not just perform it. When I returned home, I was privileged to compete and defeat the then reigning world champion in katas. I attributed this victory to my recent decision to live wushu.

Here in the Western world, students of many martial arts simply show up for their classes and, once out the door, never apply the principles they learn in class to the other areas of their lives. Living wushu means that nothing is separate from anything else—it is all interrelated.

Two Lifestyles at War

Although on the outside I seemed to have everything together, on the inside my life was a mess. I had become a father in my early teens and at the same time was recognized as a national martial arts champion, with a roomful of trophies. Having my own school stroked my ego, but because I wasn't bringing home a regular paycheck, it became a constant struggle to pay the bills and keep enough food in the house. Pride, or maybe fear, kept me from telling Master Brown about my situation.

The opposites of these two lifestyles kept me on a continually swinging pendulum. This was one of the hardest battles of my life because I was making no money from the school and was being harassed by the police when I had finally put the drug-dealing lifestyle behind me. It was at this moment that I learned one of life's most valuable lessons: it is impossible to hold onto a negative lifestyle without it interfering with, and eventually smothering, the positives in your life.

Experiencing Injustice

I remember one time I came home from a hard day of teaching, and because the crime had become so bad, off-duty policemen were walking in the neighborhood. You had to show ID to get into your own house, and I had forgotten mine at work. They wouldn't let me in. Yet I stood right there and watched a drug dealer get in without any ID. I began yelling and screaming, and a policeman came out and locked me up.

After leaving the police station the next day, I refused to tell anyone about what happened. I was angry and felt myself developing a hatred for people in authority. When I went to court, I took my martial arts portfolio to show to the judge. He laughed at me and locked me up again, using me as an example to all the people in the projects. The other message the judge sent that day was loud and clear when he let a drug-dealing friend, who had been caught red-handed with drugs, go free. This was my first time being locked up, and it came at a time when I was trying to change.

Things didn't immediately get better. On Independence Day in the projects, all the families sat in the hallways drinking beer, eating crabs, and celebrating. We didn't go to any park to watch fireworks. We had our fireworks right there, and that's what I was doing, playing with fireworks in the hallway in front of my apartment. My whole family and my girlfriend were sitting there with all the other neighbors.

Two policemen were walking the halls, telling people to turn off their music and go inside. I guess they wanted to make sure things didn't get out of hand. Well, they came over and forcefully took the fireworks from me and knocked my mom down into an unconscious state, causing internal bleeding. They hit my twelve-year-old niece and my pregnant girlfriend. Of course, I was fighting them off, and I was mad.

If my girlfriend hadn't yelled for me to stop, I think the police would have shot me to get me off them. At that point I surrendered and they cuffed my hands behind my back and ran me down eighteen flights of stairs trying to run my face into the walls.

Now outside, they were trying to put me in the police car when a crowd of people started yelling, screaming, and throwing things because they saw how the officers had treated my family and me. One backup officer told them to loosen the cuffs and stop being so abusive. On our way to the police station, the two officers told me that if I wanted to make it out and avoid them pressing charges, I needed to plead guilty. I refused and in court I was given two years probation. After this experience, I decided to go back to my old ways. I hated people in authority and certainly didn't trust them, not after an experience like this. Yet, things like this happened every day in the ghetto.

Dealing with Pain

The other thing I was hit with was my mom's death. She had cancer and it was spreading rapidly. At the time, all I could do was watch my mom decline before my eyes. All I knew to deal with this new level of pain was to use more drugs and alcohol and hurt more people. I was so angry and mean that I was treating everyone badly.

While I was going through this, I decided to step back from teaching martial arts. I stayed intoxicated day and night because I didn't want to believe that my mom was dying. On the night she died, I had been invited to New York for my first magazine cover story with Master Brown. I was so drunk that I fell asleep and missed the bus. I woke up at 5 a.m. to find out my mom was dying. This was the most painful experience of my life because she was my heart. Her last words to me, as I held her in my arms, were "Be good, Bam Bam." At this point, my world went blank and I wanted to die. The only positive thing that happened after her burial was the birth of my son, Marco, who I named after her.

Last-Ditch Effort

Somehow I had to get past Mom's death and go forward, even if unconsciously, to raise Marco. I got back into running the school halfheartedly, while selling drugs and using them myself. The one positive thing I did in my mom's honor was to host a martial arts extravaganza at the Inner Harbor. I got 7-Eleven and McDonald's to back me. It was the first time an event like this was put on in East Baltimore, and it featured top martial artists. We raised about $3,000 and donated the proceeds to the American Cancer Society.

After this event, I went out celebrating with my friends. Most people do it at a bar with beer and wine, but we did it with drugs and guns. To me, there's no difference. They all influence how you behave, and today I don't go close to celebrating this way.

It was all catching up with me. The school had moved to a better location up the street from the Inner Harbor. I said to myself, I am the Man and no one can take this from me, but before I knew what was happening, Master Brown realized I was in no shape to run a school and he closed it. On the one hand I was devastated; on the other, I was relieved to not have this obligation. I was falling apart in what should have been the prime of my career, and on the inside, I was hurt and couldn't think straight.

My last-ditch effort to pull myself together turned out to be the best job I ever had. I was hired to teach law enforcement officers for $17,000 a year, but they paid me $20,000 because of the credentials in my portfolio. Master Brown had told me about keeping a portfolio. In it, I displayed all my press clippings and certifications. It showed others and myself what I had done and was capable of doing. One more time, all the things I had done seemed to position me toward my goals.

Then addiction to a lifestyle took over and I lost everything—I had no job, no place to live, no girlfriend. The money was gone, and I had no clothes except what I had with me. I was homeless and still using drugs and alcohol. I had hit rock bottom, eating out of trash cans and at soup kitchens, living in shelters and old, abandoned buildings. Even with things being so bad, I kept my portfolio with me, worked out every day, and believed that I would reach my dream to be like Bruce Lee. My insanity was that I didn't give up the negative lifestyle, yet I thought I could do the same old things and get different results.

> You can't keep doing the same old things
> and expect to get different results.

Blessing in Disguise

My insides were at war. This lack of stability and inner peace caused me to be overwhelmed by the external distractions, and my choices led me deeper into the world of drugs and crime, ending in my incarceration. Maybe you would look at these consequences as being the worst thing that could ever happen, but I don't see it that way. For me, it was a blessing in disguise because it gave me time to spend in contemplation and meditation.

Think Before You Act

One of the most valuable lessons I learned was to think before I act. Everything you do has a consequence, some positive, some negative, and everything has side effects. If you don't follow through with the requirements, you'll never succeed.

> Think before you act; everything you do has a consequence.

Through incarceration, I learned that you should, to paraphrase Reinhold Niebuhr, be willing to accept the things you can't change, change the things you can, and identify the difference between the two. This was quite a change from my outlook as a teenager. It took soul-searching and leveling my pride, ego, and image. Once I dealt with these things, however, I experienced for the first time a clear state of consciousness—I had a spiritual experience. No, I didn't see a burning bush or hear voices, but I did have a feeling of peace and contentment such as I've never had before. I knew in that moment that the Universal Creator had a plan for me, and all

I had to do was be open to doing the next right thing in my life and He would take care of the outcome.

This change on the inside revolutionized my whole attitude toward life, my fellow humans, and the universe. At the core of my being, I knew that the Universal Creator had entered my heart and life and commenced to manifest things I could never do for myself. The rewards were well worth the struggle, because the improvements that took place have withstood the test of time.

Free Yourself from Negativity

I have always tried to use anything negative as a stepping-stone to something positive. This helps me get free of negativity, which I'm convinced will destroy me. A familiar symbol in martial arts is the yin-yang. One half is white, the other is black. Yet inside the white half is a tiny black dot, and inside the black half is a tiny white dot. This symbol represents that in all nature there is positive and negative, yet within the positive is the seed of the negative and vice versa.

This concept demonstrates the need for total balance of energy between everything in the universe—active and passive, male and female, day and night, light and dark, and so on. It is believed that when you are sick or something unfortunate happens to you, it is because your yin and yang are out of balance at some level. Therefore, when you feel pain or suffering, it is time to examine what's going on in your life, where the cause of your pain or suffering started, and how to realign your direction with the laws of the universe. I have been practicing this for a long time, and it helps me tremendously when something bad happens in my life and I'm trying to find that little speck of good that will come out of it

Respect Everyone, Worship No One

Another revelation was the importance of respecting everyone, regardless of who they are, but not worshiping anyone. I used to put people like martial arts masters, lawyers, politicians, and even corporate executives on a pedestal, but too many I've known turned out to be crooks. Now I know that when you're looking for true leaders, you should look for those who walk the walk and don't just talk the talk. They can admit if they fall short and don't claim to know it all. Too many adults talk a good line, but their actions don't match their words.

When this happens, kids of any age can spot it right away, and they watch what you do rather than listening to what you say. How many parents do you know who tell their kids not to drink or smoke while they're having a beer or puffing on a cigarette? The same rule carries over to people in authority. You can't talk bad about someone, then expect your kids to respect that person. If you want to be a leader, your actions must match your words, because kids will do as you do, not as you say.

Leaders always make sure their actions match their words.

My Pursuit of Do

This is the way of the Do, the holistic way. To achieve improvement in the world, first must come improvement in the home, the character, and the heart. Likewise, Do is the manifestation of the total being, which is struggling to maintain balance, not extremes.

Because everything in the universe is required to improve, Do is something I apply every day in my life. Being in jail taught me how to research, evaluate, and educate myself by looking closely at my negative choices and my positive traits. I learned that every action has an immediate reaction. I could have continued to make bad choices. Drugs, sexual abuse, and bad behaviors are common things in jail too. Instead, I learned to become one with my environment and make it benefit me. I realized that everything I was to do in the martial arts had to have a purpose that was universally connected to the ultimate goal of martial arts, which is self-development. I found many books to read on spirituality, good character, and history. I also worked out two times a day for two hours each time, and I tried to associate only with individuals who were positive and working hard to stay that way.

For me, being in jail was a place of higher learning, and without it, I wouldn't have had the time to get to know myself. It's a place that separates the men from the boys. I used to think that when a man was insulted or felt disrespected, the solution was to take a stand and fight. I learned to redirect this type of male macho bonding.

I learned to apologize for the negative part I played in any encounter, and for me, that's what being a man is about—being able to say I'm sorry, I don't know, or even to cry and be emotional. All my life, I tried to be the person I thought people wanted me to be. That's what I thought I had to do to get people to like me. By doing this, I nearly lost myself. Now I know that people might have liked me, but they never respected me. I've learned the hard lesson that I have to be true to myself first. Then others can like me or not, but I will be doing the best I can with the gifts the Universal Creator has given me. I hope I will become what He intends for me to become.

My pursuit of Do is more than a duty; it's my choice. I regularly share my experience, strength, and hope with others, which allows me to continue growing along spiritual lines. Having had a spiritual experience, I know that I wouldn't be the man I am today if I hadn't gone through the positives and the negatives. What goes around, comes around—the ultimate meaning of Do. I believe that everything happens in the Universal Creator's universe for a reason. The thing I was missing was spirituality.

Moving Forward

To reestablish myself in my career and reconnect with my family was hard. Everyone in the martial arts world had ideas about what had happened to me, but it was all based on rumors spread by those close to me. To move forward, I had to have a

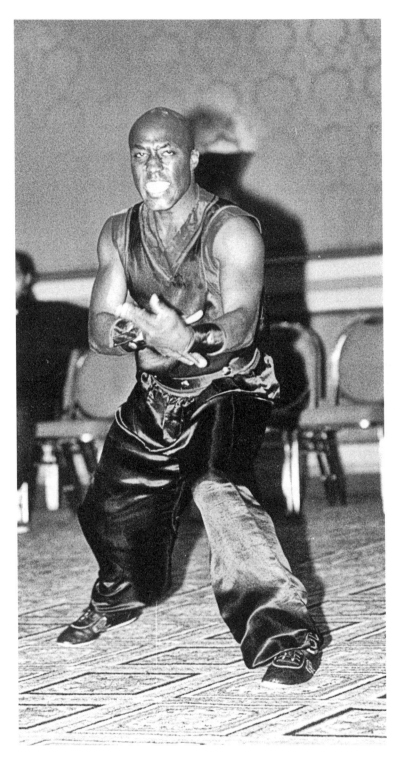

The first few competitions that I entered after being in jail were nerve-racking. Focus and determination helped me keep my cool and perform well.

childlike honesty about my experiences and share them with those I felt a need to be truthful with. By letting others know what I had done, and what I needed to do to stay on track, I thought the whole world would remind me if they saw me going down the same path again.

I remember my first tournament after being incarcerated and getting my job back with Master Brown. We drove to the Top Ten Nationals, a karate tournament in Atlantic City, New Jersey. I was very nervous. The next day at 6 a.m., before the tournament, I walked out of our hotel and began my day with prayer and taiji training. Someone yelled, "Hey Willie Bam," and when I turned around, I saw it was a competitor named Rocky Derico, who remembered me from the old days. He said, "It's been a long time, Bam, and I'm happy to see you back." What a feeling I had at that moment.

As I walked back to my hotel room, the world champion at that time, Richard Brandon, came up to me and said hello as we embraced in a manly hug. He told me what was happening on the national circuit and asked how he could help me get back on track. I began to think that maybe everyone wasn't staring at me and whispering behind my back, but the closer it came to my event, the more nervous I got. All I could think of to do was practice my taiji breathing. It must have worked because I was able to develop a peaceful state as I entered the weapons division, and I won third place, fourth in forms.

I was elated. Then people kept coming up to me and saying, "Congratulations. I remember the last time I saw you compete, you took first place." I don't think they said it that way, but that's what I heard. Everyone was feeling sorry for me, and because I was always at my best when people count me out, it fueled me to push harder. I think I'm like a warrior who refuses to lie down and die without giving it my all.

The next tournament I went to was the U.S. Open Karate Championships, which I had won before. An amazing event happened. Everyone was there—all the champions of the past and present. It felt like a homecoming. One champion who stood out was George Chung, a man I used to train with in my early days. George took me around, introducing me to everyone and telling them about how good I was. I was speechless with appreciation, and my self-confidence needed a boost like this. That day, I placed third in forms and fourth in weapons, and I went home committed to train harder.

When I was incarcerated, I read an article Billy Blanks wrote in which he said if you train like a maniac before an event, you won't have to worry about how you'll do. How you train is how you'll perform. All of a sudden, I was ranked in the top five.

About this time I began writing to magazines and had the courage to call editors and speak to them directly. I remember one of them saying, "You were in jail at one time, right?" I said, "Yes, sir." He said, "Well, we don't do articles on ex-cons, because once we put one on the cover of our magazine and he went right back to jail." I felt uncomfortable for a while after that. I thought about the things I had done in my life, good and bad. I knew I had gone through the stage when I thought I was a product of my environment and used that as an excuse for my behavior. All that thinking did was hinder my growth and limit me. In jail, I had learned that, no matter what, I am a child of the Universal Creator and always will be.

In the end, it was a blessing in disguise, because I have been featured inside and on the cover of this editor's magazine and probably every other martial arts magazine published in this country today. I am currently writing a monthly column for one. I have achieved many things, but they don't determine my success. I measure my success by my ability to stay true to myself and to contribute to life in a positive manner.

Today I feel like a newborn child, one who has built a foundation on honesty, open-mindedness, and faith. Through universal harmony, be it physical, mental, or spiritual, I have gained understanding, strength, confidence, control, and awareness. When any of these attributes set in, you must be in tune with them to flow into the right choice at the right time. These are principles I believe in and teach in my curriculum called wushudo, which means flowing in harmony with the universe. Daily practice of wushudo is helping me and others to develop as balanced individuals. Then maybe someday society and humanity will be balanced. At least it's a start.

2

Universal Principles

The key to self-development lies in concentrating not so much on what you need to change in the world but on what you need to change in you.

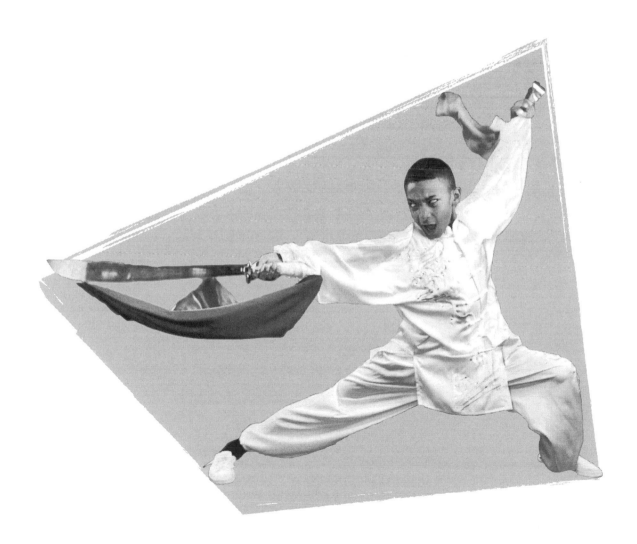

Your success in becoming a balanced individual is in direct proportion to your willingness and ability to grow and change. It is essential to learn, train, think, research, experience, and discover while you constantly explore yourself inside and out. Only when you become secure can you begin to see and feel your self-development. Life is about discovering, through positive and negative encounters, your limitations on physical, mental, and spiritual levels, then finding ways to go beyond these limitations.

Achieving this level of understanding calls for honesty, open-mindedness, and a willingness to take a searching and fearless look at where you have been, where you are now, and where you want to go.

Sometimes I find it hard to make the right choices, especially if it seems as if the whole world is trying to pull me in the wrong direction. At times like these, I step back and reflect on how far I've come. I think about where I grew up and the life experiences I've had. I read old articles, look at old pictures, listen to music with lyrics that remind me of the bad times, write articles about what I remember, or go back and visit places that have bad memories. Regardless of what's going on in my life, I find a way to fit this into my schedule. I've even taken a day or two off from work to go through this process. When I get to the other side, I always learn something about myself and am ready to move forward.

Although it takes three important principles—honesty, open-mindedness, and willingness—to reach this level of awareness, it also takes several other characteristics to help you progress in your journey toward self-development. These include patience, persistence, righteousness, unity, charity, sobriety, courage, self-denial, and love. Adopting these principles will not only help you attain and maintain self-development, but will also allow you to reach a level of peace with yourself and others.

Wushudo

Before describing each principle in detail, I will present the great design that these principles belong to. Wushudo is an expression of martial arts meaning to flow in harmony with the universe. It is a vehicle to help you on your journey through life—a road map for developing physical, mental, and spiritual fitness. Don't mistake wushudo for a new form of martial art. It's just a name for an individual's approach to self-development. In fact, wushudo doesn't adhere to one system or style of martial art, but it encourages freedom of self-expression. The twelve universal principles that exist at the heart of wushudo are meant to strengthen whatever martial art foundation you now have, or, if you aren't a martial artist, to enhance your personal travels through life.

Ideally, you will be able to flow through life with little resistance to what each day brings, but of course you will be tested. Just at the moment you feel you are spiritual and on the right path, challenges always occur. What you do in the midst of this conflict, however, determines how far you've come and how much further you have to go. If you do fall short, the answers are right in front of you, but you have to make the correction and do your very best not to make the same mistake again.

> What you do in the midst of conflict reflects
> how far you've come and how far you still have to go.

Recently I had a parent-student meeting at my school and the subject of undelivered equipment orders came up. I quietly explained that the items had to be custom-made and that was the reason it was taking so long. Still, a few parents and students loudly confronted me with their dissatisfaction in front of other people and tried to make me feel guilty. I was embarrassed because I felt they were deliberately trying to put me down, and I felt hurt at their unwillingness to understand that I saw the problem as unavoidable, at least on the school's part. I did my best to handle this situation with diplomacy and respect. On the inside, I was in turmoil. I needed time to process what had just taken place, and I felt at high risk of venting my frustration toward my students. Because that is something I refuse to do, I asked a couple adult black belts to teach the following two classes. The last class of the day was for black belts only, so I got a chance to work out with them as we engaged in full-contact sparring. Afterward, I felt better because I was able to vent my frustration with a good physical workout.

The lesson is that, because I was able to control my emotions and remain respectful, those individuals and I have been able to move beyond ignorance to improved relationships. This never would have happened if I had gotten angry or defensive. It was a sign of maturity for me. If we constantly go through life causing friction or engaging in negative behaviors, we will never experience the beauty and joy of the moment and our chance for peace and happiness, which are natural by-products of the way of wushudo.

Beyond Styles and Systems

There is no single way or single system for developing the self, just many concepts that have great effectiveness. Any system is useless if it develops clones, because then you will only meet limitations. I tell my students not to try to be just like me. Each of us can learn the same techniques, but we must develop them in an individual manner. The truly effective system is one that brings about the freedom of internal and external expression, and wushudo is designed to do just that.

Although associating yourself with one system or style of martial art can give you a feeling of identity, the downside is that in real-life situations you may find yourself with a false sense of security. When it is time to stand alone—not for fame, fortune, or recognition—you can literally fall flat on your face! This is because restricting yourself to one style of martial art constrains your abilities and deprives you of your creativity, spirit, and virtue. By closing yourself off to other styles and systems, you are limiting your knowledge and ability.

Although it is difficult for anything outside of a system or style to receive positive support, comfort, or direction, if you strive to go beyond the structure or individual

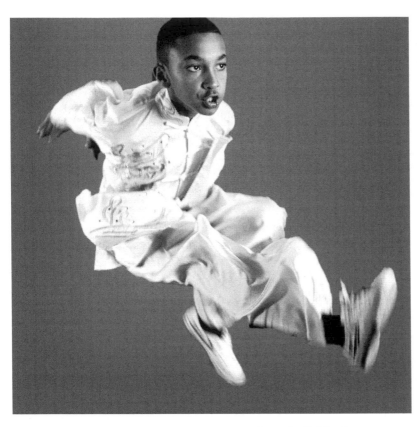

The highest level of martial arts training allows individuals to perform with total freedom of self-expression.

style, you will be able to flow and grow with everything. When you demand respect and honor while maintaining discipline, confidence, focus, and enthusiasm, you'll be able to reach past the boundaries of a specific style. You'll surpass all limitations.

Way of Wushudo

In fact, when you think about it, the highest level of martial arts training is to be able to perform beyond all boundaries, systems, styles, and techniques with total freedom of self-expression. Remember, you can achieve this only after you have developed a strong foundation in a particular style or system.

When artists paint pictures of what they see from within, you see all the details and beauty of what they are trying to display, and every time you look at it, you see something you didn't see before. If a martial artist in motion is captured on film or video, you can see the same thing. This is the raw purity of expression, and it is something that martial arts should support and promote, rather than stifle it within the limits of a rigid system.

Therefore, my wushudo curriculum allows each individual a way to find their inner purity by tapping into those attributes that shape and enhance all techniques. For example, when you're able to use such things as fluidity, grace, power, speed, and balance in harmony with your body movements, they will personalize your punches, kicks, blocks, flips, katas, and self-defense techniques. This helps you function beyond the boundaries of styles, methods, systems, and organizations and gives you freedom of self-expression.

By itself, wushudo doesn't make you great. Rather, you are successful only when you learn to make the principles of wushudo work for you through self-expression and continuous harmony with all situations. With total commitment to the universal principles introduced in this chapter, you can begin to demonstrate the effectiveness of this system.

There are several negative situations that will test this commitment, however. The world is full of people who are suppressed by racism, government, schools, jobs, family, friends, or other things. Any negative force that holds people back creates a selfish, aggressive attitude and makes people want to fight with others, intoxicate themselves with chemicals, or die.

To combat these harmful tendencies, your goal, according to the way of wushudo, is to flow in harmony with everything in the universe, and to accomplish this you must find some way to become balanced physically, mentally, and spiritually. Balanced human beings can bring about a balanced society. Many people have forgotten that they were born to live in the world and, instead, let the world live in them. Said another way, they succumb to worldly values instead of universal principles. Making more money, buying a bigger house, or accumulating earthly possessions simply doesn't make people happy. Remember, we said earlier that happiness is an inside job. You have the strength to make your environment better by doing the Universal Creator's will to the best of your ability.

One way to accomplish this is to focus on changing your shortcomings rather than pointing a finger at others, judging them, or trying to direct and control them. For example, you must choose to fight only for the cause of righteousness. This is the true meaning of self-defense. There is nothing you can offer that is more precious than good character. Therefore, if you choose to fight because you are a mere brawler, a selfish and aggressive person, or a vainglorious bully, you deserve the highest expression of disapproval because this displays bad character.

The primary focus of wushudo is developing the self. Our training focuses on controlling ego and diminishing selfish, aggressive, brawling attitudes, among other character defects, by staying in top physical condition and practicing basic punches, kicks, stances, footwork, grappling, throwing, tumbling, strength training, cardiovascular exercises, equipment drills, and kata and weapons routines. When you practice these techniques a thousand or more times, one of these character defects is bound to surface, and when you push through it, you show growth.

For instance, when performing a kata, you should be able to express the bounties of joy, happiness, and self-confidence in all movements, demonstrating your inner peace. Therefore, the most important aspect of training and fighting, whether it is full contact, freestyle, point sparring, or any other type, is to stay humble and have a calm mind. In this state you will properly place your techniques; you will be in control of yourself in the fight and stand a better chance of winning.

This is the Way of Wushudo—the individual self-expression of flowing in harmony with the universe, unrestricted and free to unite as one with natural, universal laws. My instincts cry out against being bound to a particular style, system, concept, or method, and my life experiences have taught me that truth is outside of any fixed pattern, because styles, systems, and methods are only partial truth. You'll only have 180 degrees of knowledge instead of the full 360 degrees—the full cycle of life. There again, if you get hung up on the cycle, you'll lose personal expression, the way that got you there.

It's about the ability to use all ways and be bound by none. Whether it be a tool from the urban jungle, Bruce Lee's system of jeet kune do, muay Thai, Brazilian jujitsu, Chinese gongfu, Korean taekwondo, Japanese karate, boxing, or wrestling, I borrow from many sources to enhance my ability and the wushudo curriculum. Things that we have added will always be incomplete because of our policy to remain open to new knowledge, yet complete because we strive to perfect whatever is at hand

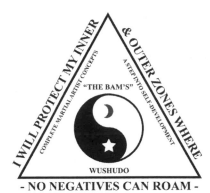

and naturally flow to the next stage. This is what I have been doing all my life, and it was my ability to do this that helped me live through the situations I've been confronted with. When I was in jail, I realized I was adapting to my situation and not reacting by harming myself, as I had said I would do if I were incarcerated. This was when I started to understand what wushudo is about.

Wushudo Symbol

The wushudo symbol, representing universal wisdom, visualizes the concept that knowledge is a never-ending cycle, with no beginning or end, but continuous, just as a circle. It is not for us to worship, but simply understand, because wushudo teaches us to worship only the Universal Creator as our higher power.

The pyramid stands for the house of knowledge and is divided into three parts: the left point stands for the past; the right point stands for the present; and the top point stands for the hereafter. Looking into the pyramid, you see 360 degrees of knowledge. This is what the yin and yang symbols represent as they fit together like pieces in a puzzle. Inside the dark, negative side is a light star, and inside the light, positive side is the moon. As you can see, within every force, whether positive or negative, there exists the spirit of the Universal Creator and our focal point.

Humans can create many things but can never duplicate the stars and the moon. Look closely at the wushudo symbol, and you can see that all knowledge for self-development flows as one, and anything that stagnates you is wrong for you. You must flow in harmony with the universe, just as the wushudo symbol flows inside the pyramid of knowledge because this is one step to self-development.

Understanding This Approach

Violence in America has been present in every generation—from the Wild West to the Roaring Twenties, from the baby boomers, to Generation X. No group is exempt. Today, with the escape into alcohol and drugs, individuals from all walks of life and every economic level are committing many crimes. Addiction is half of the problem, but the other half is the lack of a principle-centered lifestyle.

People who build their lives around the seven deadly sins—pride, greed, lust, anger, gluttony, envy, and sloth—often become egotistical, conceited, and self-seeking. This can lead to selfish pride without justification, which is spurred on by conscious and unconscious fears. Humble people can accept pride in knowing they did something well, but self-important people pump themselves up because they are afraid to fail or appear less than others. Pride is the breeder of most human difficulties and the chief roadblock to progress. It lures us into making unrealistic demands on ourselves and others—demands that we cannot meet without preventing or misusing our universal God-given instincts. These negative demands encourage us to focus on universal principles such as honesty, patience, and love, which are the foundation of wushudo.

Of course, we all have traits such as pride, anger, and envy to some degree—they're a natural part of our development. It's when we take them to extremes that we get into trouble. For example, when I go all over the world talking about my struggles, I take pride in sharing the lessons I've learned. When things that other people do bother me and I feel mean, I have a right to be angry as long as I react responsibly and appropriately.

Anything that does not flow naturally with this universe is in opposition to universal principles. Wushudo teaches us to accept life at face value, meaning that everything is happening as it should be, according to the Universal Creator's plan. Nothing, absolutely nothing, happens in this world by mistake. I had to accept where I came from and what happened to me and set goals about where I wanted to go before anything else was possible. Only when I accepted life completely on life's terms did I find peace. Today I concentrate not so much on what I need to change in the world as on what I need to change in me. In the concept of wushudo, if you don't have this attitude, followed by positive action in your daily life, it's hard to have purity in what you do and achieve individual growth.

Training Philosophy

In 1970, I began studying various forms of martial arts and other physical contact sports, including kenpo karate, judo, taekwondo, jujitsu, pa-kua, taiji, wing chun, Kang Duk Kwan, northern Shaolin, Death Ke-do, universal flow, Chinese wushu,

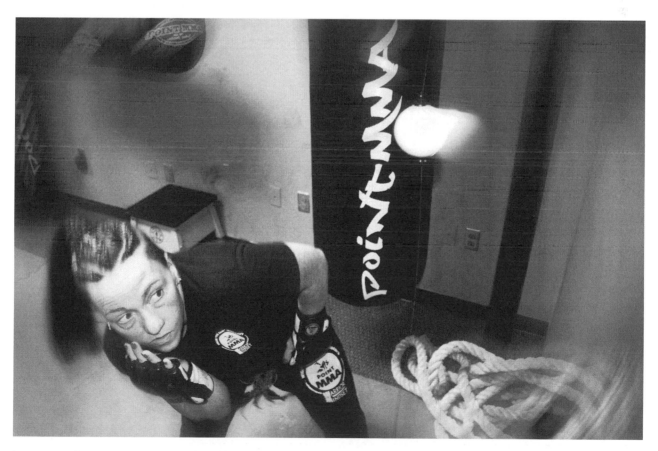

In a quest for constant self-improvement, I incorporate something from everything I study into my martial arts curriculum—from kenpo karate to boxing to gymnastics.

boxing, wrestling, gymnastics, and street fighting. Something from everything I studied has become part of me and manifests itself in an expression that focuses on fitness, forms, weapons, self-defense, and self-understanding.

My most serious studying and training took place while I was a student of Master Dennis Brown. He has helped thousands of students rise from some of life's worst conditions through studying gongfu, which has helped them live life on life's terms. Master Brown taught me that martial arts develop people not only physically but also mentally. If you allow the training to invade your spirit, you will improve in several ways, such as earning better grades in school, being recognized through job promotions, and leading a productive life.

> If you allow martial arts training to invade your spirit, you will lead a more productive life all around.

I introduce my students to traditional and modern techniques with an understanding of a spiritual way of life. The traditional builds good character, something our society is lacking today, and the modern shows us how to stay involved in change. When we add this to the wushudo principles, students are able to demonstrate self-expression and freedom of movement rather than robotic responses.

The process works by taking free-spirited individuals and choosing for them the proper techniques and responses. Then allowing them to grow and eventually to flow back into the free, unstructured form they came from. It is important to help people maintain their sense of humor, creative expression, spontaneity, and child-like honesty so they can continue growing.

Training is diverse yet satisfying enough to suit the needs of each practitioner. It delves deep into the martial arts, beyond the superfluous tricks and gimmicks, unfolding physical, mental, and spiritual self-development. It becomes a tool enabling us to reach our full potential as human beings. We are, after all, no more than what we contemplate.

However diverse and unrestricted the training is, it still requires putting forth 110-percent effort into executing techniques. Your skill can then bring about fluid mobility with a minimum of effort and, at the same time, maximize your penetration of targets and goals. Nonfunctional techniques are absent. Your techniques efficiently use the basics, selecting the best form from the arts, borrowing what is functional, and storing away what isn't useful.

Wushudo is an infinite progression of personal evaluations. Its ultimate application is overcoming negative conflicts. The practice of wushudo, without ever using it to harm others, is the goal of a competent student. Individual fighting skills, though advantageous, are secondary to the benefits of proper conditioning and excellent health. Versatility is what this martial art addresses, not showing off or proving individual worth.

As a youth, I tried to show off both in and outside of martial arts, and many people got hurt. I remember when I was a bodyguard for a friend who sold drugs. Another friend who worked for the man I was protecting said something bad about our boss and bragged about how tough he was. Payback time. One night we sneaked

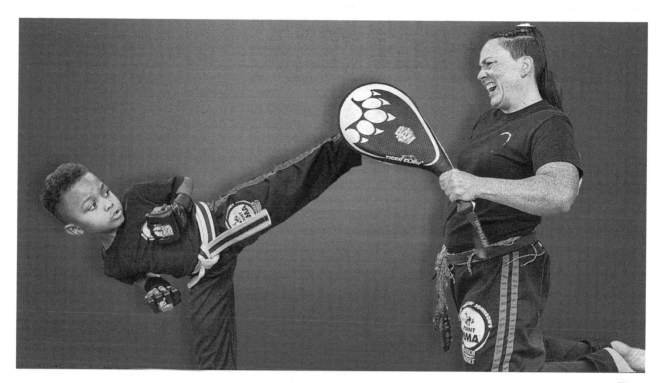

The best way to achieve continued growth is by teaching others.

up on this so-called friend and beat him up with our bare hands, baseball bats, and so on. We told him to report to work the next morning and he did.

I have always loved a challenge, but regardless of how tough or manly I thought I was, I know today that a true martial artist is humble, yet not weak; proud, yet not boastful.

You are always involved with inner competition and self-improvement. Your greatest challenge lies in overcoming the weaknesses and limitations within yourself. A physical defense against a deadly attack is a way of defending your inner peace and demonstrating self-control, which gives you enough strength to control any situation.

> Your greatest challenge lies in overcoming
> the weaknesses and limitations within yourself.

I work hard to stay at peace with myself and the world around me. As a school owner and teacher, I deal with people from all walks of life, and sometimes its sounds like they are talking down to me, like I'm some poor, dumb ghetto kid. I always listen respectfully to what they say, but I stand strong and firm for what I believe while maintaining good character. At this point in my life, I don't care if people think I'm weak or a push-over. I'm going to stand up for my beliefs and values and never allow anyone to hurt or abuse me again. This is why I work so hard to keep the old me under control—because he was crazy, irresponsible, and the list goes on. The truth is, no one can hurt me as much as I have hurt myself.

Once you come to this understanding, the only way you can keep what you have and continue to grow is by helping others. Good teachers never stop absorbing information but continue to advance as they are guided along the path of enlightenment. Think of your teachers as your guides, giving you direction from their experience. It isn't their goal to have you worship them as the master of all truth and knowledge. A good teacher simply wants respect and support, as you both share the quest for a goal. When the appropriate time comes, each must share and help the other grow in maturity, while being there to support the other until each can stand alone. Then together you can celebrate success.

Master Brown taught me this. He was a man who helped me up from the slums, and after I'd earned my second-degree black belt and won a few championships, I thought I was better than he was. I talked bad about him, claiming my way was better than his was. I even stole from him. Regardless of what I did to him, he always welcomed me back and believed in me, even when everyone told him not to help me.

The loving traits that Master Brown has for all people are the ones I strive for today. This loving quality is what makes him a master instructor. He used to say that when the student is ready, the teacher will appear. I thought he meant some person with tremendous strength would magically arrive. Instead, the teacher he was referring to was that inner voice from my conscious awareness of right and wrong. When I was finally able to hear the teacher, I had the ability and caring to make the right choices or deal with the consequences.

Universal Principles of Wushudo

I offer the universal principles that follow as a foundation for your personal journey of self-development. You are free to use them on your own timetable and at your own speed. When you embrace these principles, you will have a new approach to studying and building your martial arts path. As I and other students of wushudo can attest, you will see nothing but progress in your growth and, at the same time, you will be at peace with yourself and others.

Before you start your journey, I ask for your commitment to a belief in a power greater than yourself—a power of your choosing. I ask you to promise to guard yourself from evil forces, not only outside your ego but also within your ego. Always treat other people the way you want them to treat you. This is our duty to ourselves and to humankind.

The principles of wushudo number twelve and, simply said, are the heartbeat of self-development and support your ability to feel comfortable expressing yourself openly and freely. They are your compass as you begin the adventure of "to thine own self be true." You are not to make this trip by yourself, however. You must take the Universal Creator of your understanding with you as the driver. Go along for the ride and stay open to growth in new directions. Let go of old ideas and step out on faith, leaving your destination in the driver's hands. When I did this, I found that the Universal Creator had a vision and game plan for my life that was far greater than my wildest dreams.

Honesty

Honesty: 1. fairness and straightforwardness of conduct; 2. adherence to the facts, sincerity; 3. implies a refusal to lie, steal, or deceive in any way. (*Merriam Webster*, 9th ed.)

Being honest means that you must be willing to speak from your heart and tell others what you know to be true from your experience. Stick to the facts as you know them, and instead of telling others what you think they should do, share only what you have done in similar circumstances and in the hope that they will receive positive results. If people ask your opinion about something you have had no experience with, tell them so. Don't lie or try to deceive them, and don't make up answers to impress them. I find it best to come from a base of sharing from my experience, strength, and hope.

> Being honest means you must be willing to speak from your heart and tell others what you know to be true from your experience.

When I was incarcerated, I had a counselor who ran a group called "Who Are You?" He was an ex-drug dealer who never got caught but had turned his life around and become a prison guard and counselor. In his group, he listened to what you had to share, then cut through the tough-guy attitude and told you who you really were. He was the only man I ever met who knew when I was lying and told me so in words I could hear. Any time he suggested something to me, he could cross-reference it with the Bible or another spiritual book. I remember sharing my wushudo notes with him, and he told me, "None of that matters if you don't stay honest." Outside of a few martial artists, he was the one guy who earned my respect.

The day came for me to go in front of the judge, and I knew in my heart that I was not going to lie and would accept my consequences; I deserved them. The judge asked me how I pleaded, and I said, "Guilty, sir," because I knew truth needs no support. Then an amazing thing happened. When I was sentenced for that one year, for the first time in my life I felt free and worthy of going on with my life. My insides felt great. Telling the truth had set my soul free. I was maturing and had taken responsibility for my actions, regardless of the consequences.

Always make sure your actions and words are in agreement with who you are on the inside. Then you can live with yourself, look at yourself in the mirror, and like who you see. For example, are you someone who puts a quarter in the newspaper stand, then takes two papers? Do you think this is all right because no one saw you? Don't forget that the Universal Creator saw you, and your conscience will carry this guilt, causing you to put out negative energy. When your outsides and your insides match, you will feel balanced. Then you will be able to live with who you are and not go through life apologizing.

Open-Mindedness

Open-mindedness: receptive to arguments or ideas: impartial. (*Merriam Webster*, 9th ed.)

An open-minded person is able to take encouragement and criticism. If you are serious about developing this attribute, don't speak on matters you have no knowledge about. Listen to what others say; then research all suggestions. Keep an open mind to discover ways to move beyond your stagnation points.

Remember, your goal is to look for those things that can enhance you as a person. It is likely that you look at life from one point of view or direction, so it is important to train yourself to be receptive to new ideas. Because it is impossible to know where the message will come from, or from whom, you must at all times be open.

For example, suppose you meet some people who are beginners in a field in which you have years of experience. Your ego may tell you that you know everything and they know nothing. Wrong! Sometimes my most valuable lessons come from those who are learning—those who have not become so caught up in self that they have closed their minds to new things. Begin to go through life with an open mind and you will hear things, see things, and learn things that bypass people who are narrow minded, conservative, and intolerant of others' opinions. You will find a different world opening for you; your horizons will broaden and your perspective on life will expand.

As a student, you can learn valuable lessons simply by listening to your instructor and keeping an open mind.

Willingness

Willingness: 1. inclined or favorably disposed in mind: READY; 2. prompt to act or respond. (*Merriam Webster*, 9th ed.)

Once you have looked at yourself, including how truthful you are, and you can approach life with a mind open to new ideas, thoughts, and perspectives, the next step is to move into action, take charge of your life, and be willing to change. Have you ever wondered why some people are successful and others aren't? Those who are successful have the willingness to take action and the courage to try suggestions and continue to grow no matter what to produce the results they desire.

> Willingness is having the courage to move into action, take charge of your life, and make whatever changes are necessary to produce the results you want.

To practice willingness, it's necessary to have faith because you are going to try something without knowing for sure what the results will be. When I was in jail, most inmates around me needed to physically see and hear whatever they wanted in life, like most people. I realized that all I had at this moment was faith that my life was going to get better. I'd had faith all along; it was just faith in the wrong things. Now I was willing to restructure my life in a positive fashion. Every day, I followed my workout and daily schedule, knowing and feeling that if the Universal Creator gave me another chance, I wouldn't blow it. If He didn't, that was OK, because I was still going to give it my best shot.

Willingness comes from your gut. I call it having a burning desire. Your belief system can either make you stand still and be afraid to move forward or push you to overcome your obstacles and motivate you to succeed. To be able to take action, you must believe that you are protected by something greater than you or anyone else can imagine—many call it their Universal Creator. Embrace this spirit and it will guide you to whatever actions are right for you.

One of my beliefs is that as long as I respect the laws of humankind and live by the laws of the Universal Creator, I can't go wrong. It is the ultimate formula for success. I must step out on faith, like a child takes his or her first steps, with the willingness to fall down, stub my toe, or lose my balance from time to time as I strive to become the person the Universal Creator wants me to be. I must have a degree of spiritual fitness to be willing to take this risk. Taking time every day to pray, meditate, and read something spiritual frees me to do the next right thing in my life. I don't mean the next big thing, but simply the next logical little step in life's journey.

For example, you get out of bed, shower and dress, eat some breakfast, take out the trash, get in your car, and drive to work. There you do your best on the job, keep a positive attitude, drive home at the end of the day, and are pleasant and polite to your family. Finally, you thank the Universal Creator for keeping your mind open and clear from the confusion of daily living and for guiding you with correct thought and positive action. In this state of mind, you show by your actions that you are willing to change, adapt, and adjust to whatever comes your way. Your spiritual self is now centered in knowing the difference between those things beyond your power to change and your willingness to change those things that are your responsibility.

Patience

Patience: 1. bearing pains or trials calmly or without complaint; 2. not hasty or impetuous; 3. steadfast despite opposition, difficulty, or adversity. (Merriam Webster, 9th ed.)

Patience is a virtue, meaning that you must take your time while never losing sight of your objective. Society emphasizes immediate gratification, telling us that taking shortcuts will get fast results. Nature, on the other hand, says things that come fast don't last. If you look for the easiest, fastest way, you won't build your character, determination, and courage, to name a few. There is no substitute for your experience— so you must be patient.

> Being patient allows you to build your character, determination, and courage while never losing sight of your objective.

Before I went to jail, I saw a movie in which people who were incarcerated were counting down the days until they were released. For some reason, I didn't find myself doing this. During my quiet times in jail, I tried to reverse all the things I did in my early days and focus my energy and enthusiasm on the moment at hand. I couldn't let my mind wander because I might have destroyed myself. Instead, I wrote a set of goals, then practiced patience in their manifestation by leaving the results up to my Universal Creator. I learned to enjoy the seconds, which led to minutes, then hours, and before I knew it, weeks, months, and a year had gone by. I would not go outside what I was doing, and if thoughts tried to interrupt what was at hand, I said a prayer, recited a creed, or stopped to meditate. This calmed me down and kept me in tune to the here and now.

In a sparring match, for example, when you try a new technique, sometimes you fail. Over and over you try the same move and each time it fails. Surprisingly, it's often better to be patient and change your approach than to change the technique. In time you will be able to embrace the move you are trying to execute and make it part of you. When you are one with the movement, you will be able to apply it in a manner that's right for you and produce the results you are looking for.

Persistence

Persistence: to go on resolutely or stubbornly in spite of opposition, importunity, or warning. (*Merriam Webster*, 9th ed.)

Persistence goes hand in hand with patience. No matter how many times you fall short, you've got to get right back up and keep pushing. Not succeeding in your attempt doesn't mean you've failed; it simply means that you haven't succeeded yet.

What you are doing is gathering experience from your actions. The lessons you learn from falling down, getting up, pushing onward, and not succumbing to the obstacles in your path are the same lessons that will help you find a way to make your present actions successful.

> Persistence is that quality of never giving up,
> doing whatever it takes to get the job done.

The payoff for being persistent is that you will learn exactly what you need to do to achieve your goal, based on a personal process of trial and error. You can listen to what others tell you to do, but only after experimenting can you find the combination that will work for you.

When I was released from jail in June of 1990, into Tiney's custody, I came home and told her and everyone else that I was going to do it this time—make my dreams a reality by opening my school, getting into films, and writing books. They had heard it all before. This time, though, Tiney came right out and said, "Stop dreaming, boy. You need to shut up and grow up." I was devastated. I had been home only a day or two and already they were trying to rob me of one whole year's worth of enlightenment. To stay persistent with my beliefs, I knew what I had to do.

There were only two people who visited me in jail: my niece, Miacha, and my son, Marco. When I told them how hurt I felt and that I couldn't stay in Baltimore if I wanted to pursue my dreams, they supported me 100 percent. Between the two of them, they came up with $20 and saw me off on a bus to Washington, DC. Within a couple hours after I got off the bus, I found a job at Burger King in Georgetown and lived in a shelter until I could afford to move out. Again, the city streets were my home, and I loved jogging around the monuments in the early morning hours. Obstacles continued popping up all over the place, but no matter what, I persisted with my daily schedule. By working the universal principles, I created a zone that was my physical body, and it protected me from negative people and things. Truly believing in these principles made it possible to persist with my positive actions; I simply refused to settle for anything less.

Righteousness

Righteousness: 1. acting in accord with divine or moral law: free from guilt or sin; 2. morally right or justifiable as a right decision; 3. of or relating to principles of right and wrong in behavior as dictated by one's conscience. (*Merriam Webster*, 9th ed.)

Acting in a righteous manner simply means doing the right things for the right reasons. No questions, no excuses! If you know it's the right thing to do, then you have a moral obligation to do it. Righteous people are those of love and compassion who exemplify the Golden Rule of treating others as they would like to be treated.

> Acting in a righteous manner means
> doing the right things for the right reasons.

Have you ever watched a bushel basket of crabs? They are so busy climbing over each other that, without realizing it, they hold each other back from getting out of the basket. Beware that you're not like one of those crabs. You've got to be the one who gives others a helping hand and not take it to heart that it's their turn to move forward instead of yours. I like to think of it as paying my dues. Everyone has their time to shine. Instead of trying to put out their candle, why not help it burn brightly? It may light your way at the same time. This is righteousness.

After getting my job back with Master Brown and making my amends to him, the plan was for me to help bring his school to a successful level, then move on to my goals. That day came, and as I was about to be replaced by a new head instructor, I was asked to warm up the students. Overcome with emotion, I asked to go to the rest room and on the way, I grabbed my things and took off. If I could have expressed my feelings without being disrespectful, I certainly would have, but I couldn't. I'm not saying that Master Brown was wrong in replacing me or that I was wrong in running off—we both were simply doing our best in a difficult situation.

Now, with no money set aside, I stepped out on faith and began to work my plan to start a school of my own. Part of me said the most righteous thing I could do was move as far away from Master Brown as possible so there would be no possibility of his students following me. I knew I couldn't live with myself if this happened. At this point, the Universal Creator stepped in and led me to a new location, not too close and not too far from Master Brown. I didn't take any of his students with me, and I believe because I was clear about my values and principles on this issue, it left the Universal Creator free to lead me in His direction. It all worked out—today I have my own school and Master Brown comes in every year to teach a seminar. I took the path of righteousness and our relationship is great.

If you are practicing righteousness, you don't push other people because of your motives or hidden agendas. You don't exhibit negative behaviors to hurt, take revenge, or destroy others. You want what's best for them, even if it means you can't move forward yourself. You have a firm belief that your efforts in helping someone else will pay you back tenfold.

Unity

Unity: 1. the quality or state of not being multiple: oneness; 2. continuity without deviation or change as in purpose or action; 3. the quality or state of being made one: unification. (*Merriam Webster*, 9th ed.)

Unity goes hand in hand with righteousness. Regardless of who we are working with, the principles of righteousness and unity ask us to set aside our differences and work together for the common good of everyone, to see our common needs and how we are much more alike than different. Unity supports the adage of putting principles ahead of personalities.

Having your own business may be the American dream, but it's a lot of hard work. Before I opened my school, I had always left anywhere I was teaching just before it was time to promote someone to black belt. I let my personal life interfere with my professional commitment. It was normal for me to focus on myself ahead of the students

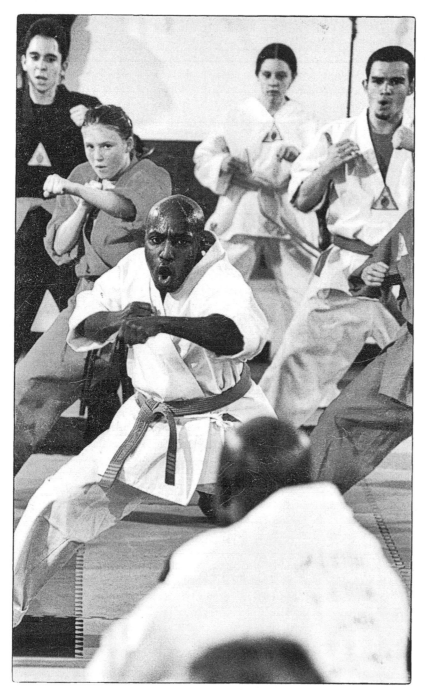

Unity, as demonstrated in group kata, allows us to set aside our differences and work together for the common good.

and martial arts concepts. Now that I had my first school and was running it as a principle-centered business, I promised myself that I would avoid the pitfalls I saw in other martial arts school owners. This meant I couldn't run and would have to find some way to keep everyone at the school united, including the black belts.

One Saturday afternoon, I was holding a kid's black belt test and two parents walked out on the floor and told me, in front of the other parents and all the testing students, that my testing method was inappropriate. Their behavior was so disrespectful that I had to postpone the test. The hardest part was that it was unfair to the students, but those two parents crossed a line that we couldn't recover from at that moment. Of course, we are long past this now—it was just painful at the time.

Every test I've run has had its challenge, but the principles keep everything in order. That's why I put them in my life and into the business: they protect me from me. During these challenging times, I sometimes want to respond disrespectfully, but I know it would destroy the possibility for unity. So I bite my tongue and focus on the overall goals.

As individuals, first we must focus on developing our own abilities and attributes. Then we can hold hands and encourage each other to achieve individual success. Once we each become strong, we can work together to build strong families and strong teams. Individuality without team support is nothing, and team support without individual expression is of no use. The great Michael Jordan is a living example of this. Being a brilliant individual player helped him take the Chicago

Bulls to a level of success unmatched in the history of basketball, because he was able to transform his individual expression into the team effort. At the same time, the team supported his ability to express his individuality.

Charity

Charity: 1. benevolent goodwill toward or love of humanity; 2. generosity and helpfulness especially toward the needy or suffering; also: aid given to those in need; 3. a gift for public benevolent purposes. (*Merriam Webster*, 9th ed.)

A charitable person is one who gives to another with generosity and compassion, and with no ulterior motives for themselves. It takes a good deal of maturity to reach a point where you can wish well for others, ahead of your self-centered goals. It's like giving a gift with no thought of getting anything in return. You do it from your heart because you want to—no recognition, no pats on the back, just the satisfaction of knowing you did the right thing at the right time.

> A charitable person is one who gives to another with generosity and compassion, without any ulterior motives.

Every year, I promote a martial arts event called the Martha Johnson Extravaganza in honor of my mother. In 1999, as I was going from business to business to get sponsorship, I continually met with people declining to contribute. I got so frustrated that a month before the event, I was ready to call it off, but I didn't. I remembered that my mom always did the best she could for me and that she wasn't a quitter. So I couldn't be either.

That year, the show was a live theater and martial arts demonstration about my life, and the people loved it. The man from McKim's, Master Brown, and people close to me talked about how special it was and that it should be showcased to youth throughout the school systems. The press even gave it rave reviews.

The money from the ticket sales and the sponsorship was divided three ways—to a local charity, McKim's Community Center, and to buying a tombstone for my mother's grave. The night was a huge success by everyone's standards, and now hundreds, if not thousands, of people all over the world know my mom.

Many times during my career as a professional martial artist, I have had opportunities to include one of my peers or students in a photo shoot for a magazine cover shot or article. It makes my heart feel good to let others have a chance to shine. I don't say this to brag; I just like to do for others what I wish others had done for me on the way up, because it makes me feel good.

Sobriety

Sobriety: 1. the quality or state of being sober. 2. not addicted to intoxicating drink: not drunk; 3. marked by sedate or gravely or earnestly thoughtful character or demeanor; 4. showing no excessive or extreme qualities of fancy, emotion, or prejudice. (*Merriam Webster*, 9th ed.)

We usually think of someone who is sober as not being drunk or under the influence of drugs. I take this a step further by saying practicing sobriety means restraining yourself from all the negatives of the world, such things as having a bad attitude or displaying bad character traits. It also refers to people who are caught up in lifestyles of lying, cheating, or stealing, and obsessive behaviors such as gambling, overeating, or being promiscuous. Living a life of sobriety means working on your negative character traits and shortcomings and constantly trying to achieve positive outcomes. None of us are perfect, but we must subscribe to seeking progress rather than perfection. This results in a state that we can describe as sobriety.

> Practicing sobriety means restraining yourself
> from all the negatives of the world.

Learning to restrain myself is the hardest thing I have ever had to do. From the beginning I was caught up in the negative lifestyle and would hurt people for just looking at me. I remember one night a group of us had been to a Prince concert. This guy started staring at my girlfriend and I went off. I ran over and began kicking, punching, and slamming him to the concrete, and when the police came, we ran. The guy was out cold and, as we drove away, I saw the ambulance taking him to the hospital.

Today, I don't do things like this because, to me, sobriety is a quality of living, thinking, and giving of your true self, which combines all twelve principles.

Courage

Courage: mental or moral strength to venture, persevere, and withstand danger, fear, or difficulty; implies firmness of mind and will in the face of danger or extreme difficulty. (*Merriam Webster*, 9th ed.)

Many people think of courage as having the ability and guts to be powerful in the face of danger, to not be afraid to fight and destroy others. I prefer to look at courageous people as those who have tapped into a special inner place and found a connection with the Universal Creator that allows them to step out on faith in a situation they otherwise would want to retreat from. Courageous people don't look for the easy, soft way but are willing to do the hard work necessary to reach their goals or confront a difficult situation. They are willing to accept responsibility for the things they need to change, then move ahead without complaining.

You must be able to recognize that everything has its own time and place, and you must have the courage to step ahead of the team and be a leader or call the team to task if members are falling short. I don't think you can tell in advance if you have courage. It's only when you are thrust into a situation by surprise and you rise to the occasion, doing what you need to do, that you display courage.

> A courageous person rises to the occasion
> and finds a way to overcome a difficult situation.

One challenge I faced came when I left Baltimore and went to live in DC. I was on parole, and one of the restrictions was that I couldn't leave the state I was paroled in. I made my choice based on a belief that I would return to my old ways if I stayed in the old environment. I knew I was wrong, but I went anyway. I simply had to follow my dreams and I couldn't do that in the old lifestyle. The immediate gratification worked. I had a life free of my old behaviors, a good job, my standing back on the tournament circuit, and my own apartment—life was good.

The day came when I voluntarily went in and told my parole officer the truth. Then I had to go in front of the judge who had sentenced me. I told the judge everything that had happened in the two years since I had been paroled. At the same time, though, I showed him a portfolio I kept of the positive achievements I had made in those two years. I admitted I had done the wrong thing but hoped that the outcomes I had achieved would count for something. At first, they both did everything they could to prove that I was lying about what I had been able to achieve. In the end, they not only said I was doing a fine job but also asked me what they could do to help me continue to turn my life around.

Someone once told me that the truth needs no support. That's what courage is about—knowing that you are standing for the right things for the right reasons and stepping out on faith that the Universal Creator will make things come out right in the end.

Self-Denial

Self-denial: restraint or limitation of one's own desires or interests. (*Merriam Webster,* 9th ed.)

Self-denial means avoiding things that are bad for you, things that are negative, and things that will give you immediate gratification at the expense of long-term rewards. Overindulgence in negative behaviors can lead to your self-destruction. Many times it is easier to see an external enemy, but the most devastating blows can come from within. Keep yourself in check in the following areas, denying yourself any of them to excess: egotism, hatred, conceit, bigotry, impatience, jealousy, self-pity, anxiety, selfishness, fear, false pride, intolerance, laziness, condemnation, arrogance, revenge, uncharity, resentment, anger, self-seeking, envy, frustration, sense of inadequacy, remorse, worry, and self-reliance.

> Self-denial involves avoiding behaviors that give you immediate gratification at the expense of long-term rewards.

I had a hard time trying to deny myself anything that I thought would make me feel good. I didn't care about the consequences—only the good feelings of the moment. The concept of denying myself anything I wanted or could get my hands on just wasn't the way I lived before my incarceration.

Before I was paroled, I went through some soul-searching and praying to get a handle on how I could change my life. One key was to learn how to deny myself pleasure of the moment in return for inner peace. I knew I could always go back and find an easier way by selling drugs, but I wanted to try a new way of life. I remember the time Tiney called and said she had just picked Marco up at the police station because his mother had left him in the house with no food for three days. Out of the blue I was faced with moving my son into my small efficiency apartment that the shelter rents to people trying to improve their lives. This was something I had always dreamed of happening, but I didn't think it would happen so fast. I had no idea how I was going to make this work, but he needed his dad and I was given custody. Somehow I was going to have to deny myself some immediately gratifying things I had gotten accustomed to and take care of Marco without losing sight of my goals. Marco and I have been together seven years, and the real blessing is that I was able to come to his rescue before he repeated the same cycle I went through.

Again, spiritual fitness gave me the courage to practice self-denial, and little by little I have developed this attribute into a working part of my life.

Love

Love: 1. strong affection for another arising out of kinship or personal ties (maternal love for a child); 2. attraction based on sexual desire: affection and tenderness felt by lovers; 3. unselfish, loyal, and benevolent concern for the good of another. (*Merriam Webster*, 9th ed.)

Almost everyone defines love in terms of a verbal expression of how they feel about someone, someplace, or something. I think it goes beyond words to an action that shows others how you feel about them. Love is also the ability to listen without judging, to help without seeking anything in return, and to receive criticism without closing your mind to fight and defend what you feel.

> Love goes beyond a verbal expression of how you feel to an action that shows others how you feel.

There is a saying: it is a fact that we have feelings, but feelings are not facts. Through self-love you learn to work these principles into your life by first stepping away from those people who are trying to direct your efforts and stifle your freedom of expression. Then you can come back in a manner that's respectful to either correct them or thank them, whichever is appropriate.

I have been able to love all people, regardless of what I feel they're trying to do to me. For example, with my father, through my new way of life, I have been able to express my love to him by bringing him to my school to teach self-defense from a street attacker's perspective and by being his son. I have accepted that my dad will never change, but I still love him. There are guys who I grew up with and did bad things with who I still love. Today, I don't approve of their behavior and choose to not be around them, but I still love them. It's much easier to love people and accept them for who they are than to hate and have negative feelings.

Being able to love a person enough to do what is good for them regardless of your feelings is called tough love. Parents often practice this with their children by setting limits. Tough love is one of those things you are apt to appreciate after the fact rather than at the time, but it is valuable all the same. Being able to express and receive love is a barometer of your inner fitness and especially your self-esteem. Love is the glue that keeps the principles together, as you work on bringing peace, harmony, and happiness into all life situations.

Unconditional love is to feel, express, touch, and care for another person and expect nothing in return. It is accepting other humans as being exactly where the Universal Creator means them to be at any time and loving them the way they are. Unconditional love is something everyone yearns for—to be loved and accepted as being all right just the way you are. Once you understand this concept, it will give you great joy to pass it along to others.

Working the principles of honesty, open-mindedness, willingness, patience, persistence, righteousness, unity, charity, sobriety, courage, and self-denial on a conscious level is displaying a love for yourself and for humankind. It's the greatest gift I've ever had.

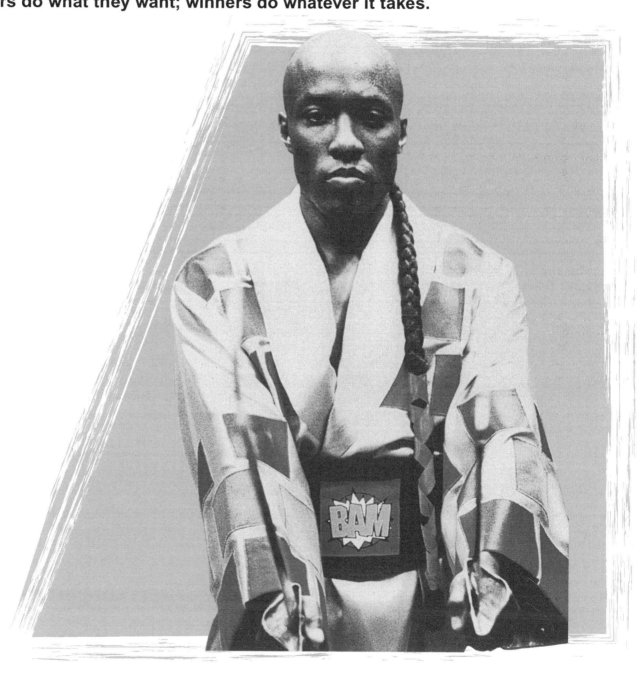

Champion Attitude

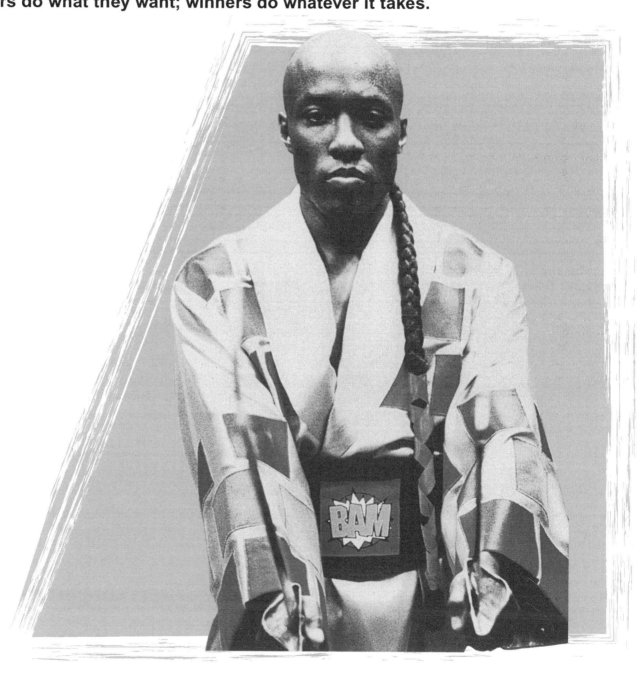

3

Losers do what they want; winners do whatever it takes.

Most people, especially athletes, go to great lengths to improve the look and condition of their bodies. They strive to keep their bodies clean, healthy, beautiful, and strong. They realize the importance of following a healthful diet supplemented with vitamins, exercising vigorously, and getting plenty of rest. If there is an ache or a pain, they consult a doctor and take medicine. Surprisingly, though, they tend to ignore the condition of their attitude. To anyone who wants to become a champion, achieve success and happiness, and live in peace and harmony, developing and maintaining a positive attitude are crucial.

Developing a champion attitude means going through a process of natural growth, with set development stages leading to a display of superiority in whatever goal you are pursuing. As a champion, this attitude is visible on three levels—how you appear physically, your frame of mind, and your connection to something greater than yourself—in other words, your total posture. This is how disciples of martial arts differ from many other athletes and people. Our focus as martial artists is at all times on total development. It is much more than a sport, an activity, a pursuit, or an endeavor—it is a way of life!

If You Can Conceive it, You Can Achieve it

The following are some definitions of attitude: a position of the body suggesting a thought or a feeling; a behavior or conduct indicating some purpose or opinion; or a state of mind. Our attitudes are outward displays of our inner feelings about someone or something.

To develop these feelings, your powers of imagination fuel your mind, and it operates like an inner movie screen. Everything your mind projects on this screen reflects in either a positive or a negative attitude. Most important, whatever you think about, whatever your mind can conceive, you can achieve. I know this to be true firsthand. All my life I've used a mind movie screen to wander from the hardcore reality I lived in. When I saw a movie with one of my heroes like Bruce Lee, Jim Kelly, or Ron Van Clief, I saw myself playing their part, not them. When I read books and magazines, I became part of the story. I saw myself as the person I was reading about and felt the feelings.

When I shared this with teachers, my parents, or friends, they laughed and said I was just daydreaming. But I continued to project myself into anything I saw or read. When I was living a negative lifestyle, I would dream of becoming a well-known bad guy, then think I really was this bad guy. When I went out to steal something, I imagined that I was one of these bad guys and could get away with stealing anything I wanted—and I succeeded. The same was true when I went to compete. I chose someone like Bruce Lee, and I was him. There was no way anyone at that tournament could beat Bruce, and I usually did win. To this day, I still do the same thing—it's just that I use this powerful tool for positive, good things.

The power to use your mind as a positive tool is already in you. You just need to know how to bring it out. One of the great literary works of the Chinese culture is Sun

Tzu's *The Art of War*. Sun Tzu said if you make your enemy your friend, then you will know his every move. Great wars were won like this. The only difference with your mind is that this is a war within you. So, to win this war against negative thoughts and actions and let the positive shine forth, make friends with your negative impulses to understand and conquer them.

Let me give you an example of how I used my mind screen to break negative cycles. When I got a feeling or craving to get high, I wouldn't act on it. First, I played the movie in my head all the way through to the end. I saw myself buying the drugs, getting high, having fun at the party, being with girls, and feeling a false sense of power. Then I watched myself coming down from this high, feeling miserable, and not being able to stop the cycle. It would just repeat until I ended up in jail, an institution, or dead. If I could make myself get to the end of the picture, I was able to choose not to use drugs.

Unfortunately, many people don't maintain a positive attitude. They let their imaginations run away from reality, creating fears, exaggerations, dramatizations, and other scenarios of false evidence appearing real. They build castles in the air. Consequently, many negative thoughts occur, they waste a lot of energy, and these feelings eventually become personality traits.

Master Brown once told me that as long as I didn't know who was going to be competing at a tournament and who the champions were, I would go in and win. As soon as I took the focus off myself and started looking around the room and socializing with the other competitors, I would get fearful, intimidated, and lose. So I started wearing headphones and playing music that reminded me of where I had come from—where I didn't want to go back to. It made all the difference.

Champions develop a happiness and heartiness about life through their powers of imagination. They know how to adjust, how to get through obstacles, and how to turn lemons into lemonade. They develop the ability to control their destiny. What motivates them? They design their own plan, embodying an ideal they are willing to strive for no matter what the odds. They realize that they have all the tools necessary for success, and they use them to go after their goals. Champions give life everything they have and then some. To achieve success and feel happy and satisfied, both professionally and personally, we must all strive to reach 110 percent of our full potential. Take to heart the expression, "The mind is a terrible thing to waste," and use this powerful tool to your advantage.

> Champions give life everything they have and then some—110 percent.

Building a Safety Zone

Your mental attitude or posture is first reflected in your overall self-esteem. Psychologists and behavior specialists believe that we talk to ourselves at an astounding rate every waking minute of our lives, using words, pictures, and emotions in these conversations. They estimate that 50 percent of what most people tell themselves is negative. The other 50 percent is split—25 percent on unfocused talk doing battle with positive talk and 25 percent positive. This shows in today's society. Every time you pick up a newspaper, listen to a radio, or turn on a television, that 50 percent of negativity is reinforced.

You have to build yourself a place, a zone, where all that exists is love, peace, and happiness that you will fight to protect. Until you feel safe, you can't be of service to anyone else. Sometimes your safe place is a physical location, and sometimes you have to retreat inside yourself. My first experience doing this was when I was incarcerated. While the other guys were gambling, getting high, and doing all sorts of wild things, I stayed in my zone. It was hard not to be distracted by these guys, but I stayed focused. I had learned on the street to keep people not in my peer group at a distance. People not there to support and help you are there to bring you down. On the street this could cause your death.

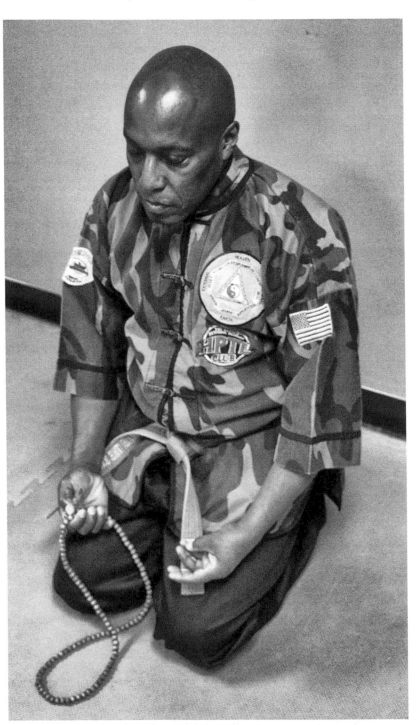

Often the kids I teach today tell me about getting into a fight at school and ask me what they can do to avoid another fight. The first thing I ask is if there ever was a time when they allowed this person to play with them, instead of waiting and watching to see if he or she was friendship material. Most kids answer yes. So there's the problem—they let the person into their zone before finding out where he or she was coming from. For me, I must protect my safety zone at all costs because it's all I have. It's where I go to take care of myself, and if I don't maintain this place, I will self-destruct and not be able to help anyone else. So be careful about who you let in close to you.

I often use meditation to "get away" and regain my focus.

Remember how the wushudo symbol reflects two sides to everything? During my first full week of incarceration, I was terrified I would die because I was claustrophobic. Sitting next to me was an inmate tying bedsheets together to escape. My mind was going crazy. I wanted to be free, but I didn't want to create more trouble for myself. I thought telling on this guy was the right thing to do, but you know what? I did nothing. I minded my business. I retreated into the safety of my mind and stayed there.

When you're dealing with your negative self-talk, you have to slow down, breathe deeply, and begin thinking about something positive in your life. Try making a list of all your accomplishments. Take time to pray and meditate. Give your problems to the Universal Creator, then sit quietly, even if the answers don't come that minute, or find someone who needs your help and get involved.

Sometimes it can be as simple as getting enmeshed in a good book, going to the movies, or watching television. For each of us it's different, but you have the knowledge of what will work for you already. It's called a gut feeling. Learn to trust it.

Adopting Champion Qualities

Qualities that distinguish great champions from the rest are discipline, concentration, and determination. They don't come effortlessly. The good news is that each of us can be a champion if we have the patience, the desire, and the capacity for realistic self-criticism of our personal ambitions. On the playing field as in life, the savvy to devise a strategy and the discipline to stick to it are essential. You must display a champion attitude in every area of your life.

> Great champions have mastered the arts of discipline,
> concentration, and determination in every area of their lives.

Discipline

In the prime of my career, I would hang out all night with my friends, then go to a tournament and win first place, but I could never win consistently or win the Grand Championship. In jail, I began to learn to discipline myself. I discovered that if you stick to your work and do your best, you forget that you're doing the same thing over and over and start to get a feeling of satisfaction from doing a good job. You'll be able to get past immediate gratification and discipline yourself to do the next right thing. This is eventually what happened to me, and my self-esteem soared.

You too can learn to make great strides in self-discipline. Start by writing down all those things you have been putting off doing and feel guilty about. Now make another list with how you can realistically complete them or do something similar. If you believe in your heart that it is something that will enhance you, then you must begin your journey to achieve it at once. Don't stop until you accomplish what you set out to do—that's discipline.

Concentration

During my last year of competing, I had to learn how to concentrate, because I felt that my race and the fact that I had left my instructor were being held against me. I knew in my heart that I should have gotten several Grand Championship calls but didn't. What kept me going was my ability to concentrate on what my purpose was. As a champion, you must have a purpose, and mine was to be an example for others, regardless of their race or position. Today, the judges, tournament promoters, and I have a mutual respect and are able to work side by side.

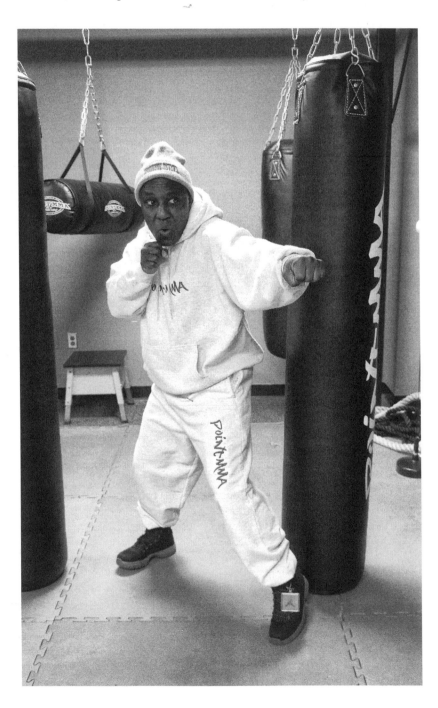

Jailhouse Workout

When I was incarcerated, I promised myself I would get in the best physical shape of my life, then go back and complete the things I had quit. I thought about all the times I had put bad things into my body and was afraid I would never be able to perform like I used too. Right then I challenged myself to train like a maniac. I had to because I loved myself and the martial arts that much.

Six days a week I worked out for forty-five minutes, starting at 5 a.m. It was a test—if I couldn't get finished by 5:45, I failed. There were no breaks, no time-outs. The more tired I got, the faster I moved into the next drill, and I did this six days a week, every week. Only on Sunday did I take a break from the physical and focus on spiritual exercises like breathing and meditation. A typical morning workout went like this:

Footwork	300 steps
Push-ups	120
Shadow punching	400
Side bends	100
Shadow kicking	400
Jumping jacks	500
Shadow kicking and punching	400
Crunches	400
Sit-ups	500
Shadow punching	400
Push-ups	120
Shadow kicking	400
Sit-ups	500
Shadow kicking and punching	400
Crunches Stretching and meditation	500

Everything I did, everywhere I went, I never lost focus on my goal to get back into shape. You might say I was consumed with this challenge. Each day I had two hours of yard time, and my activities varied. The choices were running, lifting weights, full-contact fighting, or basketball with the other inmates. At bedtime, before I made my prayers, I always did at least 1,500 sit-ups and 100 push-ups.

Do you have trouble concentrating on one thing at a time like so many people do? How many times a day do you see people driving their cars and talking on their phones and wonder if they have their minds on driving? At the office, are you guilty of talking on the phone and opening your mail or using your computer at the same time? If you are serious about reaching your goal, it is imperative that you focus on staying in the moment. Don't look back or forward even a second. Give the task at hand your total attention until you complete it, then move to the next, and the next. One step at a time, done to the best of your ability, will get you the result you are looking for.

Determination

Determination is the glue that holds discipline and concentration together. I remember at the New England Open, a national event, three of us tied for Grand Champion. I figured I had it made because I had qualified using a form I had been working on for only two weeks, and the others worked their best forms to qualify. (In this situation, you are supposed to perform something different at the Grand Championships than you did to qualify.) So, when they did their second-best routine while I flew through my usual first-place winning form and lost, I wanted to let my negative self out and be disrespectful. As I walked off the stage to the dressing room, the walkway seemed to be getting longer and longer as fans everywhere were asking for my autograph, and I knew I had to set a good example.

Boy, this was painful, especially knowing my son saw what had taken place. However, there wasn't much time for me to dwell on it because I had to turn around and do another form. It was my ability to work the principles of discipline, concentration, and determination that kept me focused on the big picture.

Remember, it's normal for many things to invade your commitment to concentrate on the task at hand. Expect it; it's unavoidable. You must have an inner determination to succeed, and no matter what, no matter how many times you may have to go back and start over to get something right, don't ever quit. You alone have control over your determination to achieve success.

Focusing on Daily Efforts

You must refocus any negative attitudes excited by the apprehension of impending danger in a positive direction. That is why it is important for you to have both long- and short-term goals. There is a lot to say for having a vision of where you want to be in a month, a year, or a decade—but not if it blinds you to the importance of what's happening now in the seconds, minutes, and hours of this moment.

For instance, there are times when I try to teach students a principle behind a technique that would help them bring forth a championship attribute. The students get so caught up in how they have seen another student perform the movement, or on getting their next belt, that they miss the point of the lesson. That is why I often remind them, and myself, that yesterday is history, tomorrow is a mystery, and today is our reality. I am impressed with the person who can focus on problems that need immediate attention, then build their successes step by step, concentrating on each as if it is the only thing that matters.

The key to getting beyond this point is to apply the principles from the previous chapter in your training. For example, when you are working on a technique and you're starting to get frustrated, you need to be honest about the situation and know that you're confused. You must be open minded by hearing and feeling your way through it, then be willing to have faith and patience. Most important, it's best to let it happen naturally. When your mind gets overly involved, you can't focus on these principles.

A champion cannot expect to make it to the top without a foundation of principles. There will always be someone, someplace, or something trying to stagnate your growth. A person more adept at the fundamentals (and therefore more secure) than you will be able to exploit your weaknesses and push you back into the pack. Focus on your daily effort in a more positive way today than you did yesterday, and it will be a stepping-stone to tomorrow.

Characteristics of an All-Around Champion

In addition to the universal principles in chapter 2, there are several qualities that champions display, not only in the martial arts, but also in their personal and professional lives.

Martial Arts

Adopting the following characteristics will improve the mental and physical proficiency so vital for success in the martial arts.

Posture: The ability to carry yourself in a positive manner, walking, standing, and talking with confidence.

Acceptance: Everything is the way it is supposed to be at any time, and you must flow with it even if you don't like it.

Self-awareness: You must always be aware of your shortcomings.

Flexibility: You must expand yourself; stretch beyond your limits; and have the capacity to adapt to new, different, or changing requirements.

Balance: Maintain a center of gravity and don't swing to extremes.

Quickness: You must respond to things quickly and without hesitation, never pausing or interrupting the fluid, natural response necessary for catlike quickness.

Endurance: Fatigue will make the strongest person weak.

Timing: Timing is the quality that makes everything you have been training to use work effectively. In fighting it's costly to be too early or too late.

Teaching: The best, and yes, the only way to keep what you have is to give it to others.

Power: You achieve power by being committed to the task at hand, with body, mind, and spirit.

Life

To become a champion, you must strive for constant improvement in and out of martial arts. Try applying the following characteristics to your everyday life.

Faith: Faith is what gives you the will to push past your limits.

Self-evaluation: You must work on your faults to become a better person.

Gentleness: Whenever you are being pushed or pulled, you must move in the same direction, contrary to your instinct to fight or go the opposite way.

Tolerance: You must become tough skinned when dealing with people and not allow your emotions to overflow and affect your character.

Alertness: You must always be prepared for life's changes, so you'll not be caught by surprise.

Perseverance: You must continue to work for what you believe in, regardless of what others say or try to do to you. When you fall down, get up and keep going.

Punctuality: You must be on time to be respected and have people count on you.

Business

Achieving professional success means keeping up with the demands of your career. It's important not to neglect one aspect of your life in favor of another. Balance is the key.

Integrity: Be sincere and honest with all people and expect the same from them.

Change: The economy is always changing and so is customer taste, so you must be in front of it. There is no such thing as standing still. You are either changing and moving ahead or falling behind.

Action: Action is always having faith that you can produce the results God intended for you. The difference between a successful person and an unsuccessful one is the ability to take action.

Adaptability: You must be able to adapt to the flow of change and commit your total being to it.

Stability: You must hold firm to the road map that works for you; don't be outside of it or distracted until it's no longer working.

Market awareness: Becoming an expert on the trends, changes, statistics, problems, and successes in your profession or industry is your responsibility. Knowing these things will help you keep on top of the competition and come out a winner.

Meeting deadlines: If you don't meet deadlines, it could be hazardous to your business. So you must push yourself to stay on top.

Following guidelines: There is no need to recreate the wheel. Just get on it and ride.

Teamwork: A chain is only as strong as its weakest link, and so it is with a team.

Financial success: The ultimate financial success comes from doing the right thing for the right reasons and letting the income generated come naturally.

The truth is that a positive thought always overcomes a negative one. This is the natural law. When the sun rises, the fog vanishes. When the light is switched on, the darkness disappears. Try turning around negative thoughts as soon as they enter your mind with a process called reformatting. When you feel angry, think love. If you face dishonesty, think integrity. If there is miserliness, think generosity. If there is jealousy, think nobility. If there is timidity, think courage.

> Focus on your daily effort in a more positive way today
> than you did yesterday,
> and it will be a stepping-stone to tomorrow.

Picture in your mind someone you are angry at, then feel how you treat someone you love. See if you can superimpose that image of love onto the person you are angry at. Give all your feelings of love to this person. Pray for them to have all the blessings that you wish for yourself, and then some. It's hard to stay mad at someone and pray for good things to happen at the same time. With some practice in reformatting, you will get successful at driving off your negative feelings and establishing a positive state of mind.

Becoming a Champion, Win or Lose

Now is a good time to point out that winning isn't the most accurate measure of a champion. Sometimes the highest caliber of champion is in the person who loses, goes back to the drawing board, learns from his or her mistakes, and takes the risk to try again. If you give your all, then win or lose, you will feel and believe that you are a champion, and you will posture as a champion.

In the world of sport karate today, I see participants who have been competing for less than a year get upset about not winning. I always was disappointed in my defeats, but I expressed my disappointments in beneficial ways by looking at what I could have done better. For me, this takes place right away by asking the judge what I could improve on, filming and critiquing my performance, and taking some quiet time to visualize what I felt went wrong. Then when I'm back in the school, those things are focal points.

A champion works at staying respectful regardless of the results, although too many athletes say that winning is all that counts and blame everyone else for their losses. One of my favorite sayings is that quitters never win and winners never quit. Realize that you were created with all the necessary qualities—honesty, confidence, focus, and control. Refuse to hold any beliefs that you were not created to be a champion. Know that you already have everything it takes to have a champion attitude. Most important, do not embrace a self-defeating state of mind—if you do, your inner self will destroy you.

Taking Action

Watch Michael Jordan play basketball or Tiger Woods play golf and you can feel their effort and efficiency in your stomach. Look at some of Bruce Lee's movies— his concentration is so intense it positively dazzles. Listen to one of Martin Luther King's speeches—the purity of intention is so extreme it is frightening. Many people say that these individuals were born with the attributes to be great. I believe that we are all born with these qualities and simply make other choices in life. Of course it would be foolish to deny that Michael Jordan, Tiger Woods,

Bruce Lee, or Martin Luther King do not demonstrate skills and strengths that set them apart from the majority. Still, there are many powerful, fast, well-coordinated men and women who are intelligent and charismatic. Merely having talent isn't enough. Positive attitude, focus, determination, and the ability to take action are the qualities that make champions. Let me say it again: if you want to be a champion you must, at all times, maintain a positive attitude, stay focused on your goal, not let anything get in the way of your pursuit, and go for it now! There it is—the secret of champions. I believe that if you talked with any champion, each would say the same thing. Champions didn't sit around and wait for glory to come to them. They got up off their behinds and took action. It won't be easy; there aren't any shortcuts. Start by embracing the principle of honesty, be willing to learn new things and change, be patient with yourself, and do a realistic self-evaluation. Don't get caught up in an overabundance of emotion, selfish desires, ego gratification, and wanting to win at any cost. Now set your goal and be realistic! Realize that you will need the proper training and a positive support system to be successful.

Self-Motivation

You've got to want to be successful for yourself, not for other people. Your friends, plain and simple, will probably lose interest in what you're trying to achieve. So, you have to be able to light a fire under yourself and keep it burning. You have to push yourself harder when you're alone than you would around others. I know this from personal experience because I never had a training partner until recently. I always trained by myself and liked it that way, because I don't like to socialize during my workouts. I also say bad things to myself when I fall short. So for me, talking and socializing get in the way of a good workout—I learn more by just going with the flow and seeing where it takes me.

When I trained at McKim's, there was no heat in the winter, and icicles hung on the windows and doors. It was cold, but I couldn't let that stand in my way. The colder it was, the harder I worked out. So when, in my last year of competing, I had a burning desire to be number one, I decided to jog through the deep snow with freezing rain coming down, knowing that my competitors were not doing the same. That year I became number one.

Devise a strategy, get a game plan, and write it down. Don't hide your action plan. Put it up on a wall or a mirror in a place where you will look at it several times a day. I tape my goals to my bathroom mirror, so it's the first thing I look at in the morning and the last thing I see at night. It is important to see that long-term goal in writing. Break your plan down into a series of short-term steps, ones that will let you see progress regularly. Customize your plan in whatever way will keep you motivated and enthusiastic. It's important to see daily progress.

> The difference between a dream and reaching a goal
> is the ability to take action.

Focus

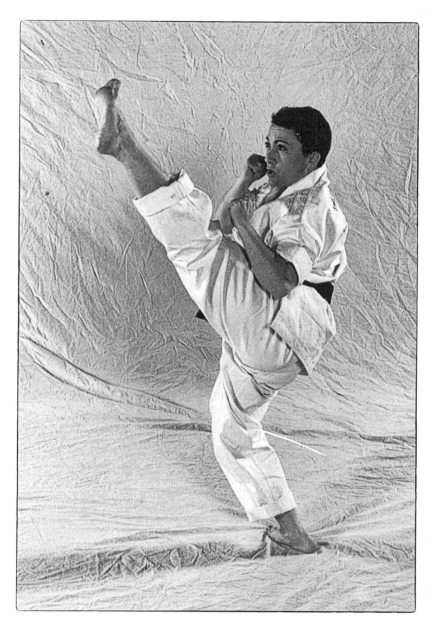

Never lose sight of doing what's directly in your path. I think of this as doing the next right thing. Champions are able to focus on problems that need immediate attention. Then they build their success step by step, concentrating on each as if it is the only important thing in the world. You cannot expect to make it to the top and remain there without a thorough grounding in the basics or without continually striving to improve. There is no such thing as standing still. You are either moving forward or falling behind. Any time you think you are getting a breather, you are really taking a few steps backward.

Given its nature, martial arts training plays an essential role in manifesting a champion attitude, because it's not just a matter of deadly fighting or effective techniques but involves a highly developed person—spiritually, mentally, and physically. Martial arts training is not simply learning something new but an expression of what has been inside

Success requires the ability to push and motivate yourself, even when others aren't watching.

you from the beginning. Don't put too much emphasis on your surroundings. When you do, you will get easily distracted and your efforts will lack purpose.

By contrast, when you are able to tap into your inner resources, accept who you are, and control yourself, you can demonstrate the champion attitude. The key here is to concentrate your focus on your inner self. Realize that your feelings change constantly—this is normal. Beware! It is a fact that you have feelings, but your feelings are only factors, not facts. They can give you a false reading because they are emotionally charged instead of being intellectually driven. Recognize that you are in control of your actions at all times. Although other people, places, and things can influence you, you have the ultimate control and power. So, put the focus on changing those things about yourself that you can change, accept those things you can't change, and have the wisdom to display the champion attitude. This frees others to search for their own pots of gold. Only then will you be able to have a positive influence on others.

Setting Goals

The following are some goals that I strive to achieve every day. I set each goal in an effort to maintain physical, mental, and spiritual well-being. They are the steps necessary for constant self-improvement. You can adopt some of these goals or alter them according to what you want to accomplish.

- Awake at 3 a.m., begin with prayer and meditation. Start your daily journey before most people are out of bed. I like to talk to the Universal Creator before I have a conversation with anyone else. This gets me grounded outside myself. I feel that the first person up in the morning has more time in the day to be productive than anyone else, so my self-esteem soars and I enter the day with an "I can do anything" attitude. I have spot-checked my spirituality. Work on my 10-Year Plan with other steps.
- Jog and work out at 5 a.m. Now it's time to wake up your body and make sure your physical muscles are finely tuned and ready to do whatever you ask of them throughout the day. At 6 a.m., prepare breakfast for my kids and wife, ready for family stuff.
- At 7 a.m. focus on where you want to go in life. Take a few minutes to think about your personal long- and short-term goals. Some of us get so caught up in the daily rat race of job or school that we forget all about enjoying the moment at hand. If you are true to yourself first, you will give your best to others.
- Plan a minimum of fifteen minutes a day to read a book or magazine that supports your self-development.
- Be committed to helping others be successful. In the process you will learn how others measure success and be better positioned for your own. This is also a real-life application of the Golden Rule: Do unto others what you want them to do unto you.
- Keep principles before personalities. Look past the person who is sharing something with you (you might not like how they look, their tone of voice, or their body language), and listen to their message. Listen to hear if what they are saying is principle centered. If it is, embrace the message and don't worry about who delivered it or how.
- Put the Universal Creator first in all things. Recognize that there is a force greater than you and give thanks every day for the good and bad things that have happened. Recognize that in everything divine order prevails.

Get started. A dream is simply that. The difference between a dream and reaching a goal is the action you take, so get moving. Now! One of my favorite expressions is that life isn't a dress rehearsal. Today is all we have, and the clock is ticking. I firmly believe that it's better to go all out to reach your goal than to sit back and say I wish I could, or if only I had. Trust me. You can live with yourself if you try, yet fall short, but to not try is the lament of the lazy and the loser.

You are the most dangerous and the deadliest opponent you will ever face! Once you understand this phenomenon, you can begin to strip away the psychological hindrances that make up your imaginary fears and replace them with the belief that you can win a particular match, perform an extremely difficult kata (form), beat a highly ranked opponent, or get a special job. Michael Jordan, Tiger Woods, Bruce Lee, and Martin Luther King are some visible people who have tapped their inner resources and manifested them into champion attitudes. If you are willing to be honest and not afraid to change, then be patient and take action, and your champion attitude will be out there for everyone to see.

Finding Balance

Remember the yin and yang concept—inside every positive is something negative and vice versa? Well, having a champion attitude has its dark side too. In the world of competitive martial arts, as with any Western sport, there are many problems that you have to deal with. The winner of a sporting event is usually thought of in hero terms—powerful, courageous, cool under pressure, aggressively on top of every situation, fearless, and so on. Yet many of today's martial artists and sports heroes have their problems, which, if you knew what they were, might completely turn you against competing.

In the past, many of my heroes spent thousands of dollars traveling the national karate tournament circuit, winning title after title, and hoping that some day this recognition would get them into the movies. At home, there wasn't enough food to feed their children. I learned from my instructor that I must take care of the home fronts of family and business first to be successful. There is a lot of pressure on you when you become one of the big names. For me, most pressure is self-imposed. The night or even the week before a tournament, I can't sleep or interact with others because I want to win so badly. Like it or not, the sport karate tournament world has become so competitive that what was once a free-time, fun activity is now a high-pressure system paralleling a profession. It's not just the performer who feels this pressure; for younger athletes, it's their parents—some of whom are living out their dreams through their kids.

For the first five years my martial arts school was open, I shielded my students and son from competing in the world of sport karate. Too often, I had seen bad character displayed by tournament leaders, and now I was seeing a shift from the principles I valued at a tournament to an event geared toward making money. My students must wait until I say they are ready to compete in tournaments, then I choose the events that I think will provide a positive experience. What I weigh in my decision is the maturity of the students and their individual ability to go into the world of sport karate and demonstrate good character at all times. I have formed a national karate team called the Better Attitude Makers, and it is our goal to be an example of what I feel athletes should be for those little fans who look up to them and ask for their autographs.

Modern sports, dominated by hard work, arduous practice, long hours learning and refining skills, sweating, bruised bones, and bruised egos, has become a job. What was once preparation for a big tournament and the anticipation of winning a six-foot trophy, your name in the national ratings, and a chance to perform in the nighttime finals on center stage for two thousand or more people has taken on the attributes of a profession. It is no longer a free-time, leisure pursuit. A role reversal has taken place.

To find balance, many superior athletes have a diversion that seems completely unrelated to the struggles of their sport. This diversion gives them time to look at things from a different perspective. My outlets are going to the movies, watching videos, and writing. Although I pursue them with the same enthusiasm that I have practicing my martial arts and staying physically fit, it puts some yin (soft style) in my yang.

Taking a closer look at sport karate tournaments has caused many people to wonder if this Western expression of martial arts has hurt the traditional values of its Eastern foundation. Remember, the original concepts of martial arts included freedom of self-expression, individual creativity, being in tune with the moment, being one with nature, and so on. Today, in many martial arts classes, students are

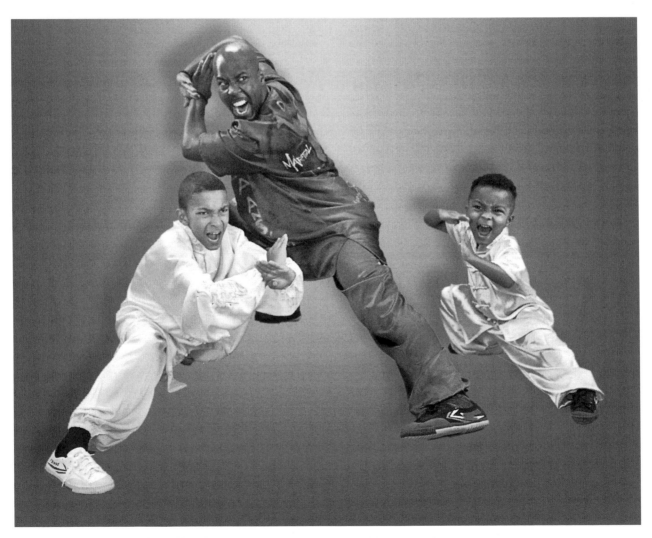

In the classroom, your focus should be on learning and improving your techniques, not on outdoing your classmates.

struggling for control over the competition mindset. In sparring matches they are trying to outdo each other to win, even when there isn't any competition taking place. They have forgotten that the classroom is the place to learn techniques and to conquer the ultimate enemy, which is self. Yes, that's correct. When it's all said and done, the only one who can defeat or beat you is you. Only through a conscious awareness of your shortcomings and character defects can you hope to achieve success. Martial arts classes provide the perfect environment for this growth, but too many people get caught in the excitement of the moment and forget the real reason they are practicing. The obvious external distractions take precedence over their internal growth, such things as social influences, hostility, fear, anger, wanting to win, showing off, and so on. A martial artist looks beyond these superficial masks for balance and a happy medium.

> The only one who can defeat you is you.

A problem many people face is that they get so wrapped up with achieving in one area of their lives that they forget everything else. Then one day they say, "Whew, I've almost got everything done, but I feel awful." They start complaining that no one appreciates how hard they've been working and get a bad case of "poor me" syndrome. They have forgotten to pay attention to something—their spirituality, family, education, material security, or a simple understanding that there's more to life than accomplishing one goal. They have created an imbalance in the foundation of their lives, which affects their self-esteem. This is how some people's marriages fall apart—one or both partners get so wrapped up in their own worlds that they forget they got married to share their lives. In short, they were willing to forego long-range goals for achieving their short-term objectives. We must break this pattern. If we don't, the result can be bankruptcy, marital problems, divorce, and problem children, as well as being physically busted up, mentally disgusted, and spiritually bankrupt.

Being able to handle pressure and making it work to your advantage will help you maintain balance and achieve success. All competitors experience a psychological and emotional response called stress, which can make or break you. It's the fear of facing a more powerful opponent than yourself or dealing with the disappointment of not winning first place. Most competitors dread this moment, and when they can't handle their feelings, they become satisfied with whatever comes. Not me, I love moments like this when everyone counts me out, and the only ones there are me and the Universal Creator. Boy, you'd better stay out of my way because I will destroy whatever is there and achieve what I'm striving for. I can live with myself only if I know I did my best.

I remember after leaving Master Brown in 1993, the national karate team I was on told me I had to attend Master Brown's tournament. I told my coach I didn't want to go. I knew Master Brown was bringing in champions and movie stars from *Power Rangers* and *Mortal Combat,* and I felt sure he would push them to win. My coach insisted, so my son and I arrived at the event.

When I saw my competitors, I said, "Let's rock this joint." That's all I could do, because I felt the deck had been stacked in their favor, and I was afraid my having left Master Brown would be held against me. So I went for the kill with no worries or regrets. When the dust cleared, I had defeated everyone he brought in. The point was not that I hadn't already beat these guys but that I had done it before I went to jail and I was the Man. Now it was their time, and I did it when I felt everyone was against me and they were at their best. This was the unconscious effort of pushing and using all the stress built up inside me to achieve success.

I think it is important for people to learn to accept their immediate setbacks and examine how they have fallen short. I always have back-up plans and other goals, and my scheduling allows me to focus on a different plan each day of the week. So when one plan doesn't manifest, I switch to the next one, or when one has manifested, I still switch to the next, because I have put my all into making sure it works.

Also, I keep things in their proper perspective, never letting the cart get ahead of the horse, regardless of what excitement or enthusiasm I feel. This usually upsets people who work with me, but I don't care how exciting things might seem, I still need my quiet time to pray on it and see it from both sides without being influenced by anyone. This is my time with the Universal Creator. More and more people are aware of the importance of living a balanced life and are looking for ways to find this balance. I think that first you must take the time to get to know yourself and be at peace with who you are. You must learn to love yourself too, even your dark, negative side. After all, you are the sum of all your parts, both good and bad. Then embrace the positive attributes of knowledge, respect, courage, loyalty, discipline, wisdom, honor, compassion, and forgiveness. Always do the next right thing, but don't ever take your eyes off your goals. If you only remember one other thing from this book, remember this: always treat other people exactly as you would like to be treated. That is the ultimate manifestation of someone with a champion attitude.

Katas and Weapons

4

You must strive to be one with the universe as you travel the path of self-expression.

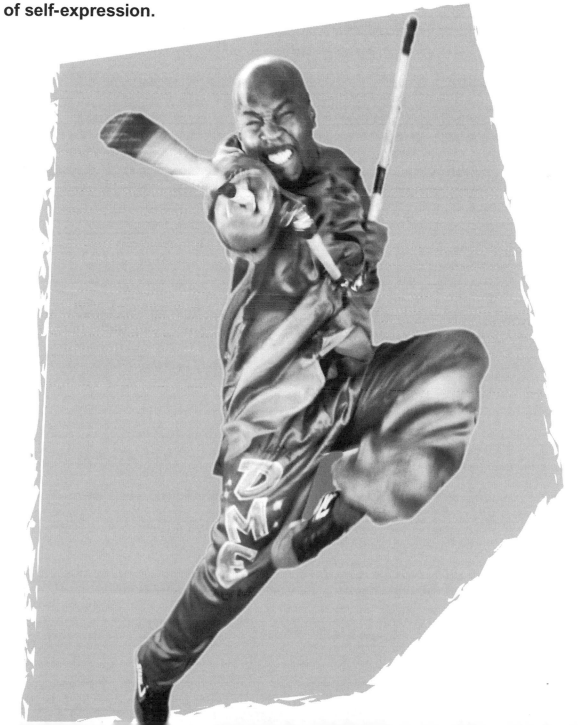

From the beginning of time, when people had to fight for survival, they developed routines to defend themselves and their families. Routines are prescribed patterns or mechanical courses of action, whether long or short, that help develop confidence and belief in your ability—a comfort level—leading to developing fluid responses, then natural reflexes in any situation. Just as in school, you learn the mechanics of writing your ABCs. Then, with practice, you develop the ability to read and write words, sentences, paragraphs, even whole stories.

Practicing katas and weapons routines brings about these feelings of confidence and instinctiveness. So when you're involved in a confrontation, either in class or on the street, your responses will be second nature. You'll be able to go with the flow and respond in a natural, effective manner that's right for you and the situation at hand.

Today's martial artists, however, are in favor of techniques; they spend so much time trying to remember every technique they have seen, heard of, or read about that they become entrenched in memorization, thinking that mastering these techniques will assure them success in tournaments and street fights.

Here's the problem. They are doing exactly the same things you're doing, so when you meet them in competition, you just exchange one technique for another, blow for blow. Both of you know the moves and the counters. Although one of you wins, the competition has all been on a technical level where you have been trading physical and mental skills.

Now, let's talk about taking these techniques to the street. What do you think your chances are of defeating an average street attacker with a prearranged set of movements? Scary, isn't it? Your attackers not only don't know your moves but also don't care. They have one goal in mind and that is to beat you down, steal from you, or whatever. They are goal oriented and have the mind-set to do whatever it takes. Your benefit from having taken the time to learn katas is that this repeated practice has developed your confidence in being able to deliver fluid, instinctual responses. You have trained your body, mind, and spirit to act as a unit, and under pressure a natural, spontaneous flow of movements will take place to whatever your attacker tries to deliver.

I'm not saying that technique isn't important. You must choose from all the techniques available, finding those that are an expression of your nature and those that you can physically execute. After all, technique won't do you any good if you can't deliver it effectively!

It's great to think that if someone comes up to you on the street and tries to grab a package from you, you'll drop to the ground and sweep him or her, or better yet, see it coming and do a fabulous jump kick that will knock your attacker off his or her feet. But if you're caught by surprise, and that's the street attacker's best weapon, what do you think your mind will have time to tell your body to do? "Nothing" is the answer. You will be left with what we call a natural response to an immediate action. There's no way you know what you're going to do. It will happen too fast. The attack will be over in a second, and you'll be lying there wondering what happened.

Basic Truths versus Learned Techniques

Knowing the difference between basic truths (natural responses applicable in any situation) and learned techniques (prearranged series of movements) can be the deciding factor in a real-life confrontation. Today, particularly in Western cultures, people are learning new techniques rather than concentrating on the basic truths these techniques stem from. People with no martial arts training who are attacked on the street will operate from a base of honest fear, and however they respond will be exactly right. The terror of the moment will put them in an instinctual, almost animal survival mode. Those trained in martial arts may pause for a second to think of what punch or kick to use. That split second could cost them their lives. Failure to know the basic attributes (in this case, honest fear) prevents them from expressing whatever technique they are using in a manner that's appropriate to their physical, mental, and spiritual ability. In a word, they are trying to work a technique instead of being one with the technique.

For example, the ABCs are the principles of most forms of communication, but we must express them in different spelling configurations and voice tonalities to be effective for the listener. If you want to be heard and understood, you must speak the listener's language. Failure to do this will not get you what you want, but when you can adapt to the moment and respond in kind to whatever is coming at you, you are going with the flow and are in harmony with the universe.

In the beginning of my martial arts training, I was so struck by every new technique I saw that my whole purpose for being was to learn the next new thing. Only years later did I realize that for all the hundreds and thousands of techniques I had in my arsenal, they all stemmed from a core of basics. For example, if you want to break someone's finger, just bend it in the opposite direction it's supposed to go!

We have to study the basics from beginning to end and not be distracted. As martial artists, the techniques we practice come into play, but only to complement our instinctual feeling for what is coming at us and responding effectively in the moment. This cannot be preplanned. It has to just happen. This is the ultimate goal I'm talking about—striving to go with the flow and be as one with the moment. When you can achieve this state, you maximize your chances of winning.

Effectiveness of Katas

People choose to study martial arts for a variety of reasons, including self-defense, physical fitness, or a desire to be a tournament champion and bring home trophies. For me, the goal was personal. I was motivated by a desire to change from the inner-city kid who made negative choices because I thought these were the only choices I had. I perceived a life as a martial artist as possibly opening the door to get out of the ghetto and into movies. Never was it my wish to be the world's deadliest fighter or the top world's forms champion; I simply wanted to feel happy and be at peace.

In my early days of training, I thought katas were for the weak guy and fighting for the warrior. I didn't get hooked on practicing katas until I was at a tournament and, just for the fun of it, I made up a kata on the spot and won third place.

Then it occurred to me that every time I struck out at the air and repeated the movement over and over, it was a form of kata. This constant repetition felt comfortable, and I got lost in the feeling of safety that came with the sameness of a movement. I also began to realize that everyone can fight, but not many people can do good kata, so I made a vow to become someone who could.

Katas combine kicks, blocks, punches, sweeps, aerial techniques, and tumbling; vary in length; and are extremely effective. They are the backbone of every successful system and have been around since our ancestors had to fight for survival.

In addition, they bring about coordination of the body, mind, and spirit. These prearranged routines develop power, grace, endurance, balance, coordination,

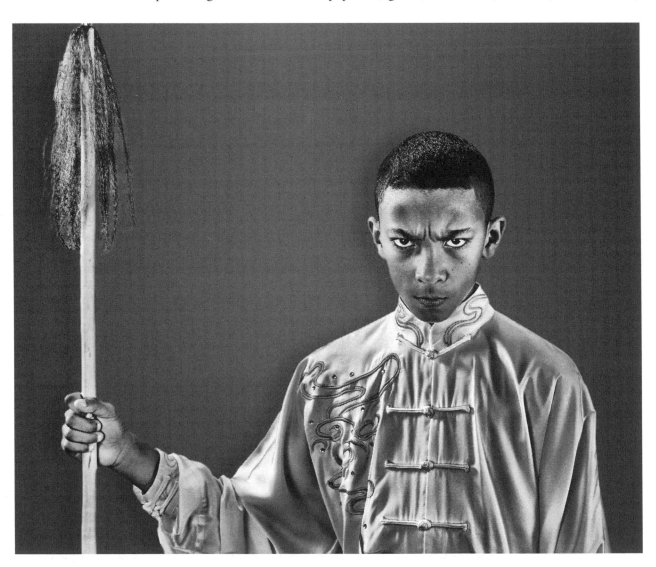

When performing a kata, strive to bring it alive using your own personal expression.

and confidence. A person must learn to be the kata, bringing it alive with their personal expression. I like to think of it as having soul. Great actors have soul. When you watch great actors perform, you forget that they are playing a part and think of them as being the person in the play, for real. Being the kata is the ultimate goal. I lived for that minute or two at a tournament when I and my kata were one.

The first katas were used to teach warriors the methods of battle. By practicing these movements over and over, they were so ingrained in the warriors' minds and bodies that the movements became instinctual. Then, when they were in a real battle, everything was second nature.

When you train, always have two or more uses for each technique, so you are accustomed to adapting it at the last minute to fit an unexpected attack. For example, you can deliver a side kick to your opponent's ribs, knee, or shin, and a round kick can smack the side of the head, back, or thigh. With a little preparation, the traditional movements will be just as effective as they ever were.

Building a strong foundation in kata training is the smartest thing you can do for yourself as a martial artist and is essential in learning any style, system, or concept. Even in such combat arts as jujitsu and jeet kune do, any series of moves you need to memorize is considered a kata, and it is the effectiveness of its application that defines its use.

In a gongfu kata, the flowing motions are similar to a medium-speed ballet dance routine. A wushudo kata has fluid, speedy motions, similar to a modern dance routine. A karate kata is slow with the focus on flexibility, power, and *kia* or *qi* (a biophysical energy generated through breathing techniques). When you examine things closely, you can see how all manners of executing katas overlap. You can call it cross-training.

Kata takes you beyond the point of fighting or brawling that happens in many schools and allows you to perform what I call moving meditation. By doing the techniques over and over again with total execution of each movement, the mind becomes detached from the motions of the body. In turn, one day enlightenment sets in. You discover total harmony of body, mind, and spirit. This is what I call personal expression: having a spontaneity to be one with self. It is one of the greatest rewards anyone can receive.

> Katas take you beyond fighting,
> allowing you to perform moving meditation.

Kata Fundamentals

There is a big difference between those who simply go through the kata movements in a robotic fashion and those who have learned to embrace the movements and enhance them with their individual expression. The defining factor is your commitment to the fundamentals of kata—those seemingly intangible attributes that, taken by themselves have little significance, but when you use them to complement your body's execution of a kata, allow you and the kata to become one.

Focus

Totally understand what's going on with every movement in your kata. Never lose sight of your imaginary opponent. Are you throwing a punch or a kick? If so, you should be looking at your hand or foot motion. If, on the other hand, your opponent is striking you, you need to have your eyes on what's coming at you. You must commit your focus to the battle at hand.

Before you start your kata, look around at where people are and identify anything, such as tables or chairs, that might get in your way. Always be aware of your surroundings, because if you get distracted, you may make a mistake or get injured. If you are totally focused on what you're doing, one with the kata, your focus isn't tangible. It just is. One way to practice focus is to stand in front of several people and throw a series of one hundred punches without becoming distracted. Add more repetitions until you are up to one thousand or more punches and nothing anyone does interrupts your focus.

You should never have to stop and start over, either because you forget what you're doing or because someone walks too close or in front of you. Stay focused on what you're doing, but don't lose sight of what's going on around you. In my first tournament after I got back from China, I had won the kata title but lost in weapons because I did a butterfly twist right into a chair someone was sitting in.

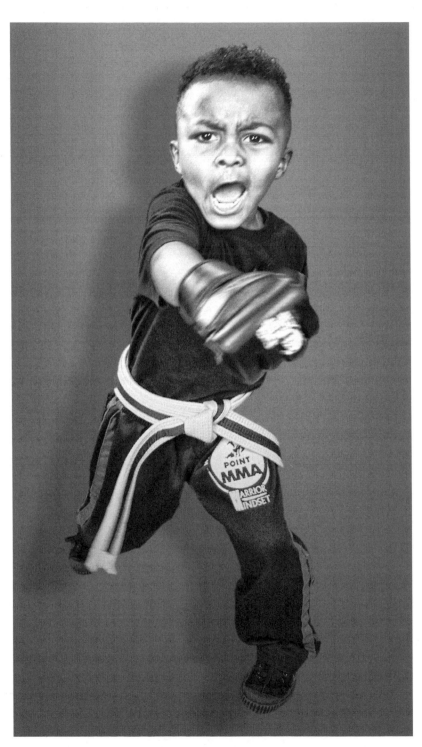

Proper breathing will give your kata power you never knew you had.

Breathing

Absolutely key to being able to execute anything in martial arts is proper breathing. The strength and power you use to deliver a technique depend on your putting your breathing behind it. When you are on the receiving end of a blow, knowing how to take a breath at the right moment will tighten your stomach and abdominal muscles so you don't get the wind knocked out of you. Proper breathing will give your kata power you never knew you had, and suddenly your movements will be explosive, especially when you accompany these moves with a rhythmic sound such as a kia at strategic points. By doing this, it will also help you express yourself throughout the routine.

Learn to make your breathing work for you, not against you, by keeping your breathing fluid, inhaling during a transitional movement and exhaling during an execution. Always breathe in through your nose and out through your mouth. To increase the amount of air entering deep into your lungs, you must learn to breathe from your abdomen, rather than just using your upper lungs, as many of us tend to do. One exercise you can do right now is to place the index finger of your right hand just below your belly button. Starting with your index finger, count down three finger widths. You have now located your Ida, source of your internal power. Make a loud sound emanating from your kia. It will be strong and powerful. Now place your fingertips on your throat and make a loud sound. You will hear a much higher pitched sound, something like a scream. Once you can implement proper breathing techniques, you will greatly enhance your endurance, timing, and concentration.

Fluidity

Picture your kata like a stream flowing toward the ocean. The stream encounters rocks, twists, turns, waterfalls, and even branches, but it has the ability to adapt instantaneously to whatever obstacle it meets. It may be forced to slow down or speed up for a few seconds, but then it resumes its rhythmic pace. This is how you should practice your kata. Choppy motions interfere with the speed and power you get from flowing movements.

Don't telegraph your movements. Slip through your transitional movements making adjustments as you need to, then the result will be breathtaking, like a waterfall.

Technique

You should execute every technique in a kata as perfectly as possible. Remember, there are no surprises here. You know exactly what's coming and precisely what you have to do. Be sure to show not only the big motions but also every little position of the arm, hand, wrist, foot, leg, turn of the body, gaze of the eyes, and so on. Make your techniques picture perfect; let the audience see their beauty, quality, and sharpness. Pause for a second or two at the final motion in a technique, holding a stance or an arm position to accentuate its importance. Making sure you fully execute your techniques demonstrates your commitment to their complete expression.

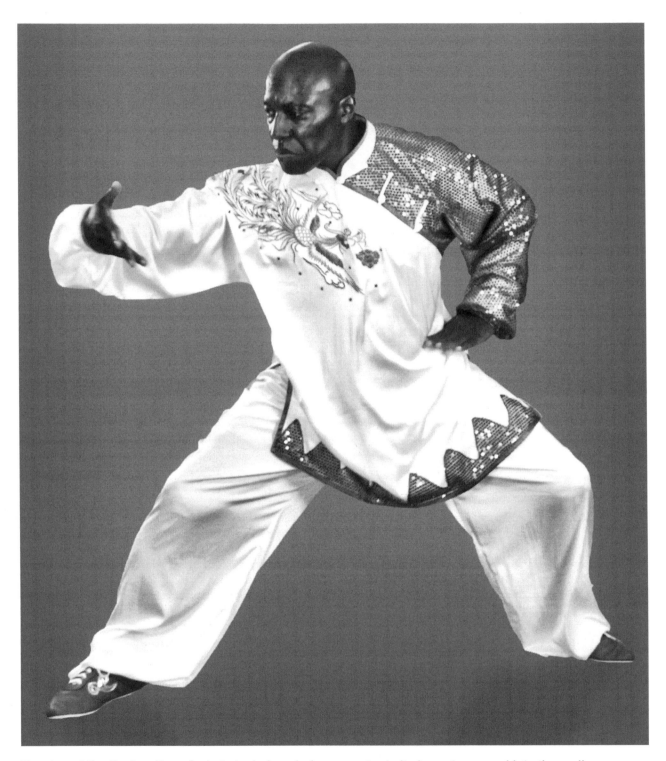

Pausing at the final motion of a kata technique helps accentuate its importance and lets the audience see its beauty and sharpness.

Facial expressions should show the emotions that you feel to accentuate the technique. For example, for a fluid, nonaggressive move, your face should reveal peace and relaxation. For a strong, powerful move, your face should look like an angry tiger lunging to destroy its prey.

Take the time to perfect your techniques. You will be amazed at what this does for your confidence and self-esteem. Ask a fellow martial artist to critique your kata and help you identify any small movements you need to clean up. Watch yourself perform your kata in front of a mirror or have yourself filmed. I make films of myself and students doing katas, first in slow motion then at regular speed, to give them something to study. It has been said that a picture is worth a thousand words. So make the ending of every technique a Kodak moment. Perhaps at your next tournament you could ask the judges what they thought about your performance and what you can do to improve it.

Flexibility

Only the young are born flexible. The rest of us have to work at it, but the degree of flexibility that you are able to train your body to deliver will be worth the effort. Flexibility is the one attribute that will complement all the other parts of your kata, allowing you to add beauty and power to your techniques because you can exaggerate them for better expression.

This lesson was brought home to me when I was in China and saw everyone outside practicing some form of martial arts at 5:30 a.m. It kept them flexible, like a good oil job on your car. If you want to keep the body running, you have to oil and grease it with exercises and movements that will keep you flexible.

Use any basic warm-up exercises, aerobics, walking, running, stretching, and so on, to maintain and increase your flexibility. Remember, if you don't use it, you'll lose it.

Body Control

The banks of a stream control the flow of the water, but in martial arts, you have to learn to control your body. Either you are in control and win, or you give that control to your opponent and lose. Body control is the one quality that separates a champion from the masses. You will never see champions execute something that doesn't fit their bodies or that they can't control. Never take something into competition until you feel confident that you have mastered the techniques. Learn what fits and feels right to your body in practice; then you will be in control of your body when the pressure is on.

Rhythm

Everything in life is based on rhythm; it's a law of nature. Just as we flow through the seasons or our daily routines, our katas must develop a rhythm that embraces all its parts and flows with our bodies. For instance, you don't usually see little kids working taiji or old folks doing flying jump kicks. It's the wrong rhythm.

I have always worked out to music and use music when I teach my classes. Even when I'm warming up before a tournament, you'll see me off to the side with my headphones on. I'm listening to music that speaks to me, and I'm getting my rhythm on. It sets my mood and gets my muscles pumping. It's an external tool to keep my mind occupied so I don't get distracted and break my flow.

Learn which songs motivate you when you're working a kata; then use them to put you in a zone where you and the kata are one. If you've never tried this, take it from me, it works.

When I went to China, my kata and weapons routines were good but not great. There, the coaches drilled me on one section of my forms for an hour or longer at a high speed and intensity. I never thought about sitting down when I got through, because then I was busy refining anything I'd done wrong. There was no music at these sessions, only the spirit and enthusiasm of the wushu athletes to push me beyond my limits. They would scream "dragon spirit," which meant to push with your qi. (Qi or kia is your body's energy source, located three inches below the naval.)

Parts to a Kata

The following are the essential parts of a kata. Mastering each part is the key to being one with the kata and expressing your true self, thereby maximizing your chances of winning.

Focus: Stay focused on what you're doing, but don't lose sight of what's going on around you.

Breathing: Keep your breathing fluid, inhaling during a transitional movement and exhaling during an execution.

Fluidity: Move like a stream, adapting instantaneously to any obstacle you meet. Your speed and power increase from flowing movements.

Technique: Take the time to perfect your techniques, doing them as perfectly as you can. It will build your confidence and self-esteem.

Flexibility: Train your body to be flexible and you will add beauty and power to your techniques. Remember, if you don't use it, you'll lose it.

Body control: Learn what fits and feels right to your body; then you will be able to control your technique delivery.

Rhythm: Develop a rhythm that embraces all parts of a kata and flows with your body. Everything in life is based on rhythm; it's a law of nature.

Kata Drills

I adapted the following drills from those I learned in China. Constant repetition will make your techniques more reflexive, enabling you to react automatically should you need them in a street altercation. You can apply the improved dexterity and confidence you gain from kata practice in your everyday life.

Slow Motion

Instead of racing through your kata, turn down the speed to slow motion, making every motion deliberate and detailed. Now you will be able to apply all parts of a kata to each technique. At first you will be amazed and rediscover details you may have forgotten, such as an exact hand position or how to turn your foot to place a kick to someone's knee.

Practicing in slow motion provides the perfect opportunity to clean up your kata because you will be breaking it down into micromovements. For instance, there's a lot more to building a car than putting an engine inside a body and driving away. What will happen when you do a kata slowly is that your rhythm will develop, and this is one of the most important things you can identify. Then after you know what you're doing and why, you can turn up the afterburners.

Section Practice

You should implement section practice only after you can increase the speed you work your kata. Divide your kata into quarters or sections of ten or twelve movements each; find a logical division. Now work each section ten times or until you have all the movements down. Then work the next section, and the next. In the end, vary your practice by mixing up the sections.

It's been said that you don't know a kata until you have worked it a minimum of one thousand times, so be patient.

Full Speed

Now that you understand sections, you can begin working your sections at full speed with thirty-second breaks between them. Focus on your balance, landing solid as a rock, and fully extending your techniques. Working your kata nonstop for fifteen or twenty minutes should put you in a state in which your heart rate has increased and your mind is disengaged. If you can work your kata while you're in this state, without making mistakes, you will not be able to remember what you did. This is what I mean by being one with the form.

You will need to have someone critique your movements and report to you. When you are able to go through your kata with speed and power, not remembering what you did, and not making mistakes, you are ready to move to another kata or perform this one on the tournament circuit.

Adding On

Katas are imaginary fights. Therefore, during your training, you can add to this imaginary situation and simultaneously incorporate all the techniques that show your true talents—high kicks, gymnastics, hand techniques, jumping techniques, and so on. By doing this, you will display your individual expression.

Don't be bound by the limits of prestructured kata routines. Take the risk to make it yours by adding the techniques that are your best.

Moving to Music

Practicing your katas to music gives you a chance to work to the rhythm of your favorite songs. Use fast music to increase your speed, slow music to check your techniques. (Note: I am not referring to practicing a musical kata, which is a form choreographed to perform with a particular song.) Adding music while you practice helps you bring out your personal flavor and adds a spiritual dimension; plus it keeps you from looking mechanical.

> Practicing your kata to music
> will help give it a unique, personal flavor.

Designing Your Kata

A good drill for an advanced student is designing your own kata. Do this by taking your best techniques and putting them together in your kata format. You can set your level of difficulty, and you can design a form that you can practice in a small space, which will improve your close-in fighting skills. This is not for a beginning or intermediate student. It is for those whose foundation is strong and who haven't taken any shortcuts in their training.

You will know when you are ready to design your own kata. It will start happening by itself; it's a natural flow.

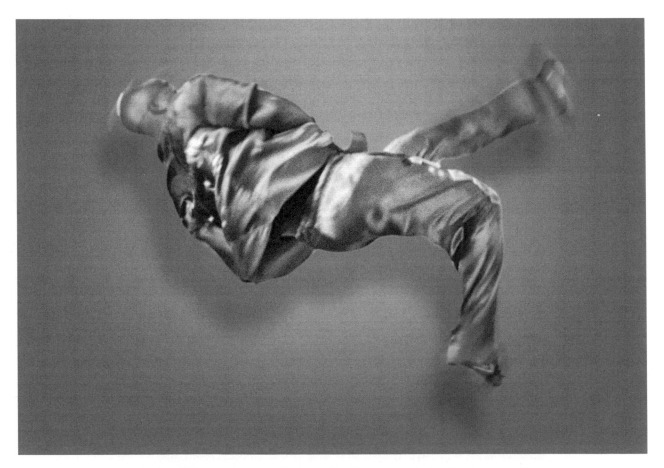

Incorporate into your kata all the techniques that emphasize your talents, like gymnastics.

Blindfolded Kata

You need a partner for this drill, or you may injure yourself by running into a wall. Start in the middle of the room with the assistance of your partner. Working your kata blindfolded helps you feel your movements and your body. Some even say that when blindfolded, they feel the form starting from inside them and flowing outward, instead of working the physical movements and waiting for them to become part of you. Remember, some fights aren't in well-lit rooms, so the ability to fight in the dark can be an asset.

Working your kata blindfolded is the ultimate test to see if you and your form are one. Try it. It's fun, I promise.

Don't shortchange yourself by thinking there is any shortcut to learning a kata. It takes a lot of time (at least a thousand repetitions), patience, and just plain hard work, but the payoff is big. You will be able to show your personal expression when you perform a kata, and you won't look like a carbon copy of everyone else. You will move from a mechanical routine to being one with the form; then you are on your way to reaching your full potential.

Weapons Practice

We often describe a person who is highly skilled in martial arts as being versatile in every category of weapons—long, short, soft, and hard. Many of today's styles, systems, and concepts have abandoned the ancient weapons for modern ones, failing to realize that if you first learn how to use traditional weapons, you have a foundation to use the new weapons.

Weapons training is an important aspect of martial arts, because the structuring of self-defense systems is the most difficult to learn. It also provides an unparalleled opportunity for uniting the body, mind, and spirit and develops control, timing, and flexibility. When you use a weapon, everything has to be in harmony, or you can injure yourself or your classmates.

> Weapons training develops your control, timing, and flexibility.

Practice using heavy weapons in a soft, flowing manner and light weapons in a strong, direct way. In days of old, martial artists used bow staffs, which were heavy, and swords made of steel or solid wood, which gave them extremely effective penetration of their opponents. Today we practice using the same heavy weapons, but we also use bamboo sticks and aluminum swords, which give us extraordinary speed and power in our routines.

Think of the yin as the yielding, internal force and the yang as the unyielding, external force. The weapon must be an extension of you, blocking, attacking, fighting, maneuvering, and evading. If you hold a weapon in your hand, you must think of and use it as part of that hand, or in a foot technique, as an extension of your foot. This is the most important thing I can tell you about successfully working a weapon.

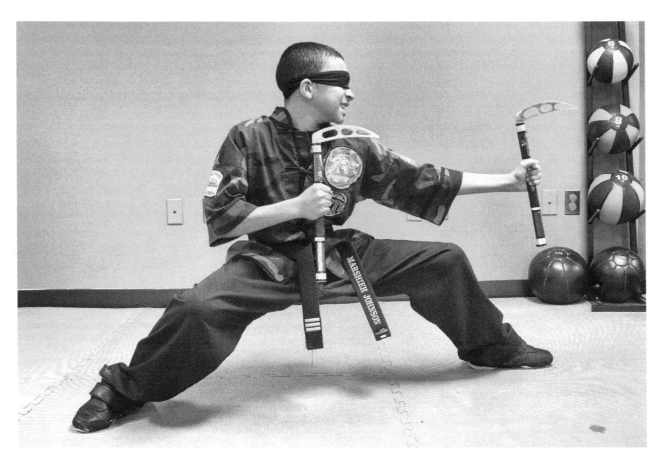

Working a weapons kata blindfolded enhances your body awareness and helps develop timing and control.

Take the time to learn a weapon kata. Mastering this technique will enhance your fighting skills, overall conditioning, breathing, movement precision, coordination, strength, speed, balance, rhythm, and most important, endurance.

Once you are confident using the kata drills previously mentioned, try practicing your weapons the same way, even blindfolded.

My personal favorites are the broad sword, short staff, spear, and double daggers. When I starred in the television series *WMAC Masters*, the director asked me to use the "Willie Bam Whip." This was a long hairpiece platted into a small patch of my hair. (If you've seen my picture, you know I'm bald. For the series, I grew a patch of hair on the back of my head that was not quite two inches in diameter.) Without my constant practice with traditional and modern weapons, I wouldn't have been able to pick up an object like this and use it as a weapon.

Effective kata training is important to developing effective skills with weapons, because how you work your hands and feet in unison determines how effective your weapon use will be. Show the spirit, rhythm, and style of the routine from the inside out. This will eventually allow you to give it your own flavor (after a thousand or more repetitions). Someday you may find yourself using one or two weapons with your hands, feet, or mouth in a manner that is effective only by making it an extension of your body.

5

Freestyle Sparring

AKA, Point MMA

Use every means possible to avoid a fight, but if it's inevitable, fight to win.

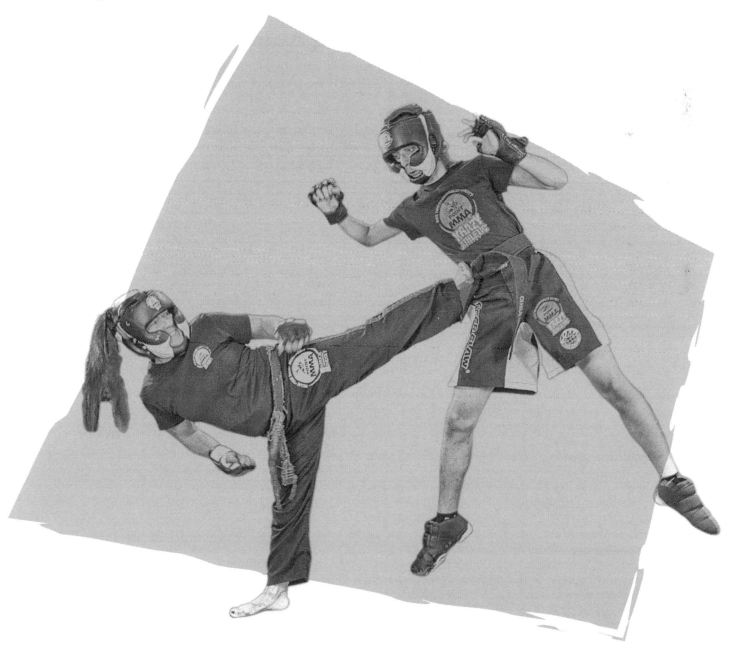

During the nighttime finals at the Baltimore Karate Tournament in 1981, one of the largest tournaments on the East Coast, it was time for the super lightweight fighting division. I had trained hard for this moment and watched my opponent out of the corner of my eye. He seemed pumped up and ready to go—it was going to be a good fight. I began easy, feeling him out, and within seconds he attacked me with a jumping hand technique to the face. My body countered, as if on cue, with a perfectly timed side kick between one of his jumping techniques. At the end of the three minutes, the match was tied four to four. My competitor had earned my respect, and I knew I was contending with a tough opponent. In the tiebreaking round, I emerged victorious, having defeated my most worthy opponent with ground fighting techniques.

The unique thing about this fight was that my opponent had no legs! Yet his skills as a martial artist weren't compromised. It was my training in universal fighting techniques that allowed me to move into his comfort zone and fight from the ground. I simply flowed in harmony with the situation, gained control, and won. This is one of life's most valuable lessons!

If your goal is to be a universal fighter, you must train in a manner that encourages all the physical elements and natural fighting techniques to come together with speed and fluidity—it's a total package. You must be able to effectively use stances, punches, blocks, kicks, sweeps, footwork, and grappling; develop them into offensive and defensive techniques; and exhibit them in freestyle sparring, in which you should also practice sweeps, takedowns, and ground fighting. Keep in mind that, although sparring partners can use all these techniques in practice and street fighting, not all are allowed in competitive sparring. This approach brings the basics you have been learning from the training floor into controlled, real-life fighting situations and gives you a chance to see what you will do under pressure. If you expect to grow as a martial artist, you must embrace all of martial arts, including sparring.

My theory of effective sparring is to understand the gates of attack (high, middle, and low), high being the head, middle being the body, and low being the legs. By becoming familiar with these gates, it will help you to execute practical, offensive moves, such as kicks to the head, punches to the body, and sweeps to the legs. When it comes to your defensive skills, watch the shoulders and hips of your opponents dip up and down. This telegraphs which hand or leg they are about to use. Control such joints as your elbows and knees with efficient angular and circular stepping to further complement your defensive techniques. Above all, your personal, instinctual ability to master and deliver offensive and defensive techniques as a natural response in any situation is what will make you an effective fighter.

Freestyle sparring is the ability to fight outside of all rules and regulations, and at different levels of impact—light, medium, and hard. It brings us close to the reality of the streets, so you will be prepared to deal with whatever comes your way. Real fighting can never be staged. It is triggered by your emotions and those of your opponent. When you are facing each other, you should become as one—just the two of you flowing back and forth—going with whatever comes with no thought process. It's strictly action and response. In combat, styles, systems, concepts, and techniques don't matter—just self-expression. Of course, if you are sparring at a tournament, the techniques executed must follow the guidelines of the sanctioned sport karate association governing that event, such as the Olympics, the North American Sport Karate Association, the National Blackbelt League, and so on.

Through freestyle sparring you develop the free mind, responses, and reflexes needed to flow in harmony with your opponent, whether in the ring or on the street. Mentally you are using everything you've learned before. Your mind is free to flow; it is in a state of not-being. It is the process of emptying your cup in order to grow, because your focus is response without thinking. When you put two people together who are responding to each other's movements, there is no time to think—just harmonious flow.

> Through freestyle sparring you develop the free mind, responses, and reflexes needed to flow in harmony with your opponent, whether in the ring or on the street.

The ability to freestyle spar is the result of good foundation training. However, I do not recommend it for beginning or intermediate students who are still developing and perfecting their basics and learning to respond spontaneously in a fighting situation. I have my beginning students start with one-step, two-step, and three-step sparring. They also learn how to execute properly delivered jabs, crosses, back fists, reverse punches, front kicks, side kicks, round kicks, angle steps, and side steps. Once you are proficient with the basics, you must be able to put together natural, basic techniques that keep you out of your opponent's range of attack. You must also be familiar enough with them to instinctively counter an opponent's move with an opposite and effective reaction—whatever the situation calls for—as in street fighting. At this point, you become a technician instead of a brawler.

When you can successfully respond with your natural techniques, light-contact, freestyle sparring begins, and you are classified at the intermediate level. The ability to focus on developing your strong points to a higher level and overcoming your weak areas is what identifies you as an advanced student. Now you are more relaxed and inclined to try different strategies and techniques, hence developing your universal fighting style.

A key factor in students' success in freestyle sparring is developing their self-control and determination. With good supervision, freestyle sparring teaches fighters to control the situation, not let the situation control them.

The science of fighting is the ability to outthink and outmaneuver your opponent—to hit without getting hit. In fighting, a good offense is a good defense. Fighters have to beat their opponents to the punch with lightning-fast techniques and quick footwork. You must attack with deception by faking to create openings so you can deliver your well-focused techniques, and you must deliver proper techniques instinctively, so your mind is free for strategy. Anyone, even national champions, can freeze in fighting situations, so use the classroom to work on overcoming this potential handicap. Remember, if you freeze in practice, you will freeze in a real fight. So beware!

> The science of fighting is the ability to outthink and outmaneuver your opponent—to hit without getting hit.

Universal Sparring Concepts

I emphasize the same combat orientation that was practiced three hundred or more years ago in my curriculum. I have simply taken the best, most effective techniques from all the disciplines to form the base of my curriculum, because it allows us to adapt and flow with any situation that may occur. Although training methods have changed considerably, it is presumed that anyone at an advanced fighting level has mastered individual punches, blocks, footwork, and kicks. The focus of the universal sparring concepts is fluidly combining these techniques and using them to execute eye gouges, foot sweeps, grabs, locks, takedowns, ground fighting, and submission holds.

I don't strive to produce point fighters, full-contact fighters, or street fighters. The goal is to bring about universal fighters—those individuals who can use all

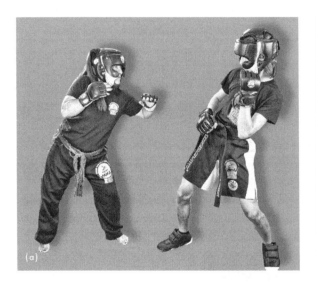
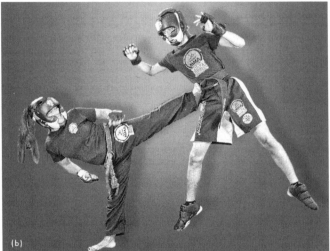
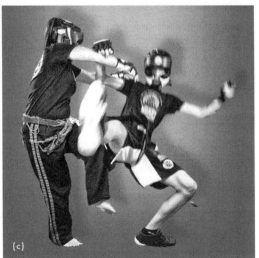

One of my favorite wushudo combinations is: (a) lead-hand back fist to the face, followed by (b) a spinning back kick to the body, then (c) a lead-leg foot sweep.

methods and approaches but be confined by none, and who can move from one technique to the next, based on their range of attack. This is a universal fighter. One early technique I drill my students on is blocking, even though most opponents are prepared to counter. We also routinely focus on combination techniques during our freestyle sparring drills. I believe that if you use combinations when you fight, one combination will surely penetrate. The basic rule for a wushudo combination is threefold—attack the high gate, face; the middle gate, abdomen; and the low gate, groin or legs.

A personal favorite is a lead-hand back fist to the face, followed with a spinning back kick to the body, and a lead-leg foot sweep. This is an effective technique, but only for advanced students.

I encourage my students to use variety in their hand techniques and footwork, including circular and angular motions, because you can't hit anything that's not there.

Deciding on what kind of strike to deliver to an opponent is usually not a conscious choice because of the time factor. It must be an immediate response to the situation. In the split second before you strike, your senses take in range, position, target, and how much time you have to react. Practice and experience are the only ways to perfect your ability to make the most effective choice when it's time to strike.

Remember to always wear safety equipment when you spar. Even so, techniques such as the ridge hand, back fist, and ax kick call for an especially watchful eye so no one gets hurt. This is the purpose of the practical sport of Point MMA. For more information on it, go to Pointmma.com

Stances

In all fighting arts, stances and footwork play an important role in coming out on top. In each aspect of fighting the stances are different. For example, the most commonly used point fighting stance starts with the individual in a short-straddle horse stance with weight evenly distributed on the ball of each foot for maximum mobility. Your front arm is loosely bent at the level of your ribs to protect your body, and your rear hand is a little higher and slightly bent to protect your face. At the same time, keep your chest turned away from your opponent to make it hard for him or her to score a point.

In kick boxing or any full-contact realistic fighting, your chest is on a slight angle for good defense response and effective offensive power.

Form the combative stand-up, on-guard stance with the balls of your feet under each shoulder, knees slightly bent, weight distributed evenly, and chest turned at a slight angle. Bend your lead arm with the elbow inches away from your lead hip and bend your rear hand so your index finger is grazing your chin.

In the proper on-guard stance from the ground, you support your body weight on your rear leg and your rear hand, hold up your lead hand to protect your face, and raise your lead leg with your knee bent at a 45-degree angle. In this stance you will be able to circle, move forward and backward, and from side to side. Your opponent is unable to know what you plan to deliver.

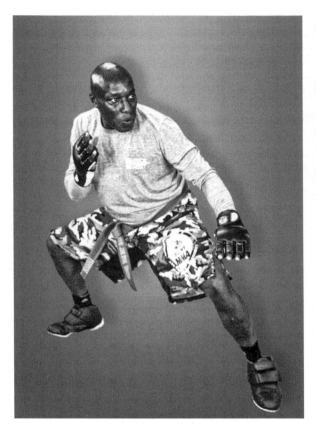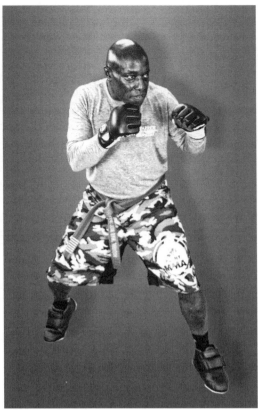

Point fighting stance. Combative stand-up, on-guard stance.

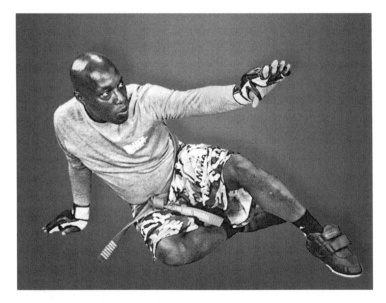

On-guard stance from the ground.

Although knowing the proper on-guard stance is essential, rolling techniques may also come into play, based on the situation. If you begin falling to the ground, you must stay so in tune to your opponent's movements that in a split second you can move into an effective offensive or defensive technique and gain control.

Footwork

Mastering the art of proper footwork is just one more component that identifies a winner. Because a moving target is harder to hit, it's to your advantage to develop footwork patterns that you can naturally flow in and out of in response to any situation. To maximize the effectiveness of your techniques, therefore, it is essential that your footwork is fluid and rhythmic, a style that fits your body type, and movements that come naturally to you.

Use the sidestep to get out of the way of your opponent's forward attack with either a kick or a punch. Simply step to the side with your lead foot as your back foot follows, and you will avoid getting hit, or when your opponent comes at you, face to face with a kick or a punch, step back to create a gap between you and your opponent's technique.

Probably the best of these footwork drills is the triangle step, because when your opponent attacks you face to face, you simply step past him or her at a 45-degree angle. Bring your back foot up and slide it past your opponent's lead foot, and just slightly in front of his or her legs for an effective, evasive technique. Follow up immediately by jamming up your opponent and launching a series of punches, kicks, or elbow strikes. Do not place your foot between your opponent's legs but use this area as a focal point for your foot placement—about twelve inches away.

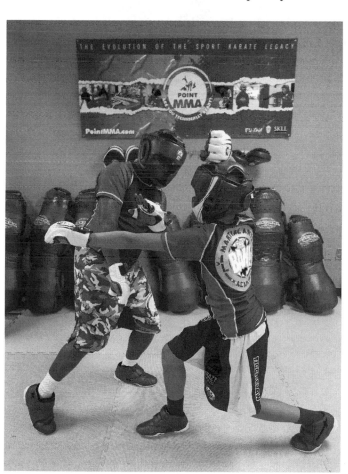

A commonly used drill from gongfu is called circle stepping, which involves keeping your opponent on the outside of your foot and never taking your eyes off him or her. Your objective is to get behind your opponent, making it awkward for him or her to function, but giving you all the opportunities you need to attack.

Creeping is taking any of these mobility drills and adding cat-like stealth.

Instead of standing directly in front of your opponent in perfect striking range, try this counter. When your opponent moves to your left, take your lead foot and step outside of their right foot in a semi-circle or half moon movement. If you always put your lead leg in the same direction your opponent is trying to go and use a semi-circle instead of a straight line, you will contain your opponent's mobility and be in control.

Triangle step.

Kicks

Kicking is your first line of defense. It gives you a chance to keep your opponent at bay with a variety of kicks, such as front kicks, side kicks, and back kicks. To be more effective, use your lead leg. There might come a time when you will be so in harmony with your opponent's offensive movements that you can get off a dropping technique, followed by an effective joint or pressure point strike.

For example, your attacker closes the gap with a straight jab, and you counter with a drop side kick to the ribs, followed by a lead-leg scissors takedown. We can also consider sweeping in this category because you must go to the floor to execute front sweeps, back sweeps, and iron broom sweep techniques. Don't forget hooking, locking, and trapping, all of which are effective with the legs, especially if your primary targets are joints and pressure points.

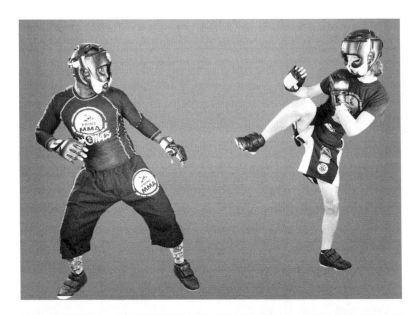

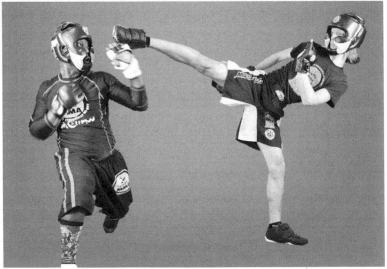

Circle stepping.

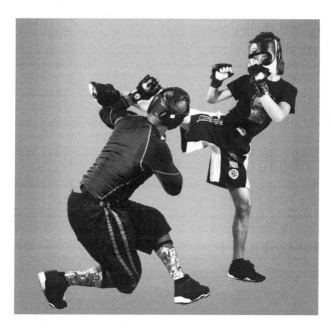

Creeping.

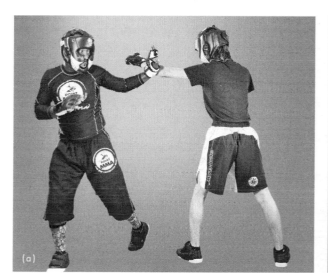

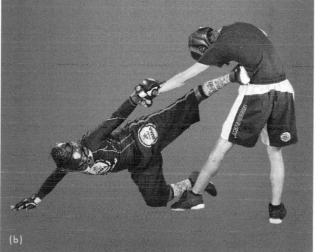

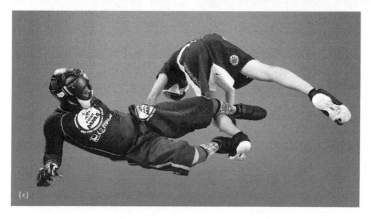

Kicking can help keep your opponent at bay. For example, (a) your opponent throws a straight jab. (b) You counter with a drop side kick to the ribs, followed by (c) a lead-leg scissors takedown.

Hand Techniques

Hand techniques are most effective on a defensive level, after your opponent gets past your kicks and comes into the punching range. Keep in mind that when you counter your opponent's techniques with your hands, follow your block with a grab and use the same hand to both block and grab. This causes him or her to feel out of control for about a half second—just enough time for you to follow your grab with a takedown or throw, accompanied by a restraining or submission hold.

For example, when your opponent throws a jab, use an outside circle block and grab with your lead hand. With your other hand, counter with a reverse punch and move immediately into a scissor takedown with your left leg across the neck and right leg across the chest into an arm bar.

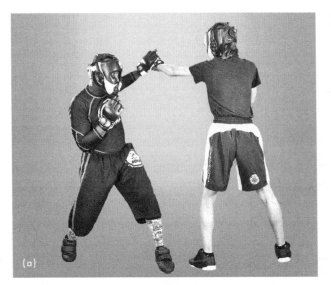
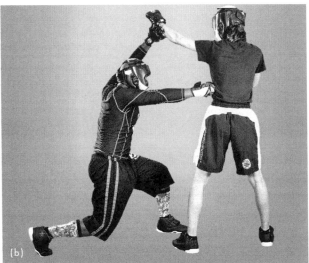
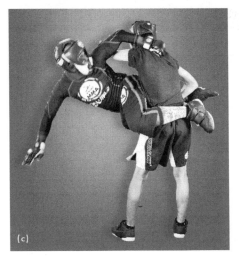
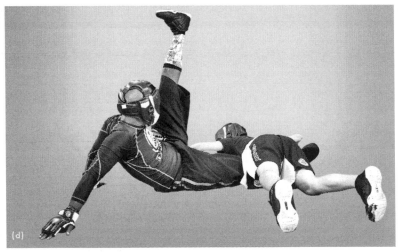

Hand techniques are most effective when used defensively: (a) Outside circle block, (b) reverse punch, (c) scissors takedown, (d) arm bar.

Takedowns

A takedown is a technique that you execute in a standing position while sweeping your opponent's lead or supporting foot, using the inside of your foot to strike your opponent's heel. You can hit the calf of your opponent's leg as well, but it requires more force. Any effectively executed takedown requires destroying your opponent's sense of balance.

When carrying out a takedown, it helps if you can grab and hold onto your opponent in some way. In an offensive procedure, lead your opponent in with a series of techniques; then use the takedown. In defense, deflect the incoming technique while grabbing hold, then taking down your opponent. Once on the ground, follow up with grappling, submission, punching, or kicking techniques.

Lead with a Jab

This is an offensive technique in which you attack your opponent with a straight jab. Follow up with a lead-leg inside foot sweep. When your opponent falls, deliver a well-placed foot stomp.

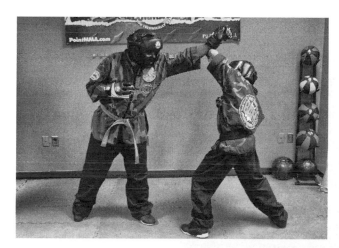
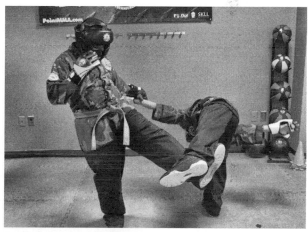
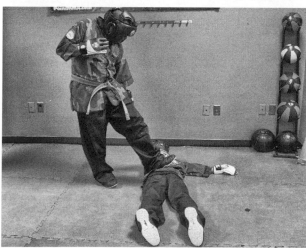

Lead with a Front Snap Kick

Take the offensive and attack your opponent with a front snap kick followed by a front sweep to the lead foot, which will throw your opponent off balance. Deliver a back sweep to the rear foot, taking your opponent down; then use a heel kick to the ribs.

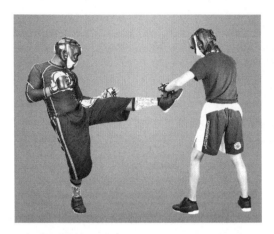
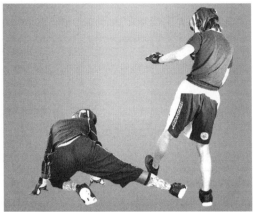
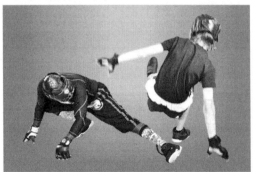
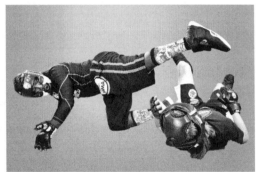

Counter a Spinning Kick

When an opponent throws a spinning kick, lunge forward, locking your arm around their calf and punching them in the face with your other hand. Now, grab their shoulder and sweep them. You are totally in control and can body slam them to the ground.

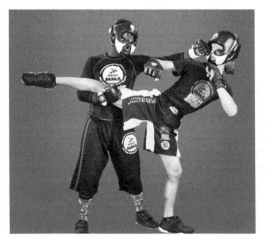
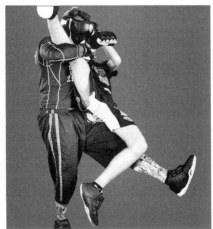

Counter a Lead-Leg Ax Kick

Your opponent executes a lead-leg ax kick. Counter with a spinning back sweep to your opponent's back leg. Then follow up with a round kick to the face.

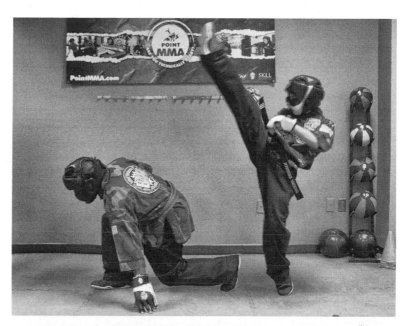

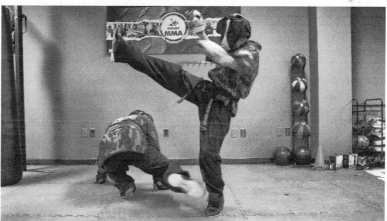

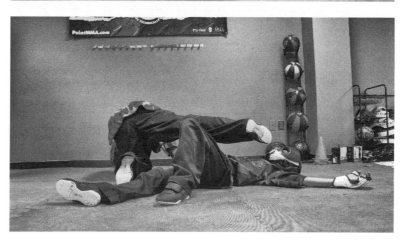

Sweeps

A technique that you use to break a person's balance by a surprise attack to the opponent's feet with your foot is called a sweep. When executing a sweep, stay close to the floor by making contact with both feet and palms for support. Do the sweep by spinning like a ball in motion. You must coordinate the body as one and stop as one to maintain balance. If you lose your balance, the sweep won't work. It differs from a takedown because you don't use your hands in the process of getting the person on the ground. However, once down by either a sweep or a takedown, follow up with a locking or a striking technique. Remember, any time you can use both your hands and feet, you pull the person's body in two directions at the same time.

Front Sweep

Execute a front sweep by dropping quickly to the ground, full weight on what becomes your rear leg and both hands. This leaves your other leg free for the sweep attack. Your

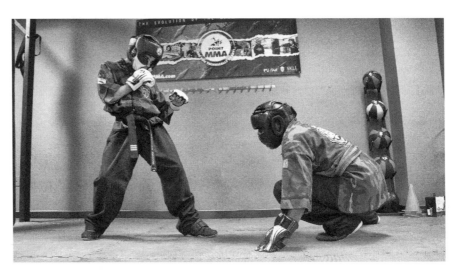

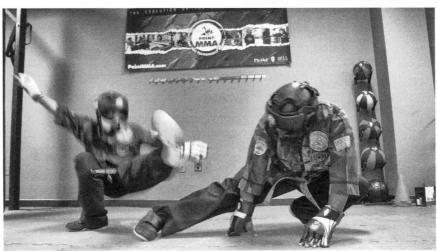

opponent can be standing on both feet or, even more effectively, kicking with one foot in the air, which gives you a split-second opportunity to make an effective counter. Again, once the sweep has your opponent on the ground, you can follow up with grappling, submission, punching, or kicking techniques.

Back Sweep

Do a back sweep by dropping away from your opponent as you put your full weight on your lead leg and both hands, leave your back leg straight. You are now able to make contact with your opponent's leg by rotating on the ball of your lead foot and swinging your leg around sharply into your opponent's leg. Make sure you keep your head moving in unison with your back foot to avoid being hit beside your head. You can execute the back sweep with a follow-up technique like the takedown.

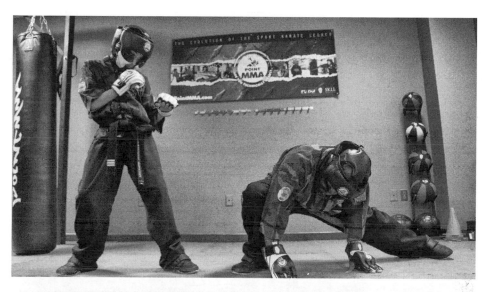

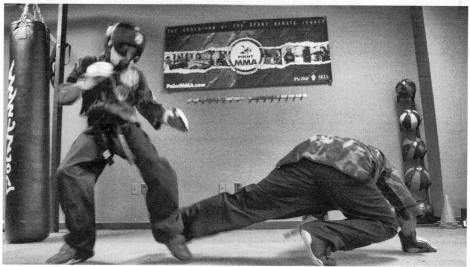

Iron Broom Sweep

A more advanced sweep is called the iron broom, and you accomplish it by dropping to the ground in a sliding motion on the outside of your lead leg and hooking your opponent's lead foot with your lead foot. Use your left hand for balance and your right hand for defense. Then swing your back leg around to cut your opponent's hooking leg from underneath, causing him or her to come down as your lead foot goes around to complete another sweep.

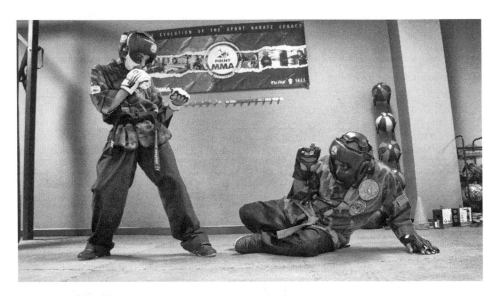

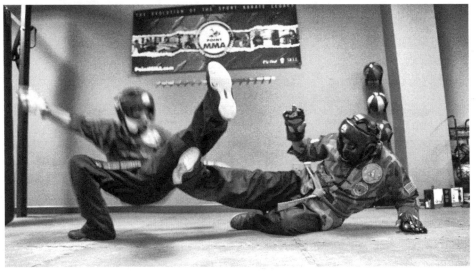

Ground Fighting

One aspect of martial arts training that you shouldn't neglect is ground fighting. Most street fights that don't end quickly with a one-strike technique but finish in a ground fighting position. Universal sparring concepts are equally balanced between stand-up fighting and ground fighting. Our approach is called top and bottom grappling, because everything you do standing up, you should be able to do just as well from the ground and vice versa.

In most schools ground fighting is not part of the curriculum. This may be partly because of the complexity involved with the body movements or because martial artists' egos tell them they won't ever be lying on the ground face up. Be sure your training includes rolls, drops, and falls to the ground. They condition the body, help you develop body control, and give you a chance to practice complex movements fluidly and realistically.

Master Kenneth Parker used to say that when you go down on your back, be prepared to kick, punch, grapple, and trap your opponent into a restraining or submission hold. Master Dennis Brown went a step further by saying you must be able to execute an effective technique on the way down. My curriculum teaches students not only to develop offensive and defensive techniques, but also to exhibit these movements in training and refine them for combat.

I got this foundation by accident in the rough inner-city schools and in street fights. It was there that my ground fighting passed the test and convinced me it enhances who you are as a fighter. Later, in the early 1970s, I trained with Mfundi Tayari Casel, considered by many to be the greatest ground fighter of all time. Easel's unorthodox style, demonstrated on the legendary *Wide World of Sports,* thrilled audiences. He proved that a skilled ground fighter has the best advantage against an upright opponent who, if overconfident and unaware of the endless countering measures available, is in a world of trouble.

Once you're on the ground, the opponent has to come down to you to launch the attack and his or her body is open, making a perfect target. You have the advantage from the ground with the right technique, and it's easier to move around on all fours. Balance also plays an important part. For one thing, balance is easy to maintain from the ground. You also have more reach with your legs, and you can use them more for jamming, trapping, and locking. Use your hands for blocking, grabbing, maintaining balance, and moving yourself about fluidly. Also use your hands for close-in jabs and punches along with trapping, grappling, and restraining techniques.

To properly execute these techniques, you must be agile enough to roll, tumble, and fall. The main requirement is to have your body conditioned to the point that it can maneuver itself into any position. Your kicking, sweeping, punching, grappling, trapping, and restraining skills must be as effective from the ground as from standing. Ground fighting is effective against one or many opponents. It is regarded more as a defensive style of fighting than an offensive style, and once you feel comfortable with this defensive way of fighting, you are ready to give your unwitting opponent a big surprise.

One of the most effective moves is to attack between your opponent's motions when he or she is extending or retracting a technique. You may counter with a leg jam to the knee or ankle, halting the attacker; a double-leg takedown into a mount; or a choke hold from a close-in wrestling move. Be adept at delivering combinations that will penetrate your opponent's defense. Go with the flow of your opponent's technique, allowing him or her to develop a false sense of security. Then, the moment you feel a weak point or an opening, launch your attack to a vulnerable area, preferably a vital spot. This will distract his or her focus and break the flow. Now you have your chance to take control of the situation.

Guard Counter

In a guard counter, your opponent rushes you from the front and pushes you backward. As you fall back, lock your opponent's hands. Then swing your left leg around to the left side of your opponent's neck and your right leg outside his or her left arm. Using your right hand, grab your opponent's left hand and point the thumb toward the ceiling. Finish by raising your pelvis.

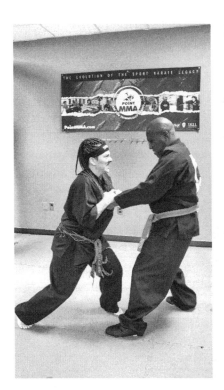 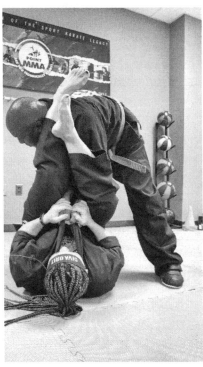 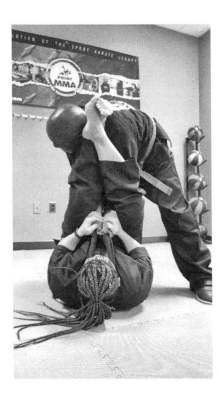

Arm Bar Counter

Another example of a ground fighting counter is to attack your opponent with a left-hand palm strike. Your opponent drops to one knee and grabs your left ankle and calf. You fall to the ground and your opponent grabs your left leg with both hands. Execute a scissors lock by hooking your right leg behind your opponent's left knee. Complete the move by executing an ankle lock on your opponent.

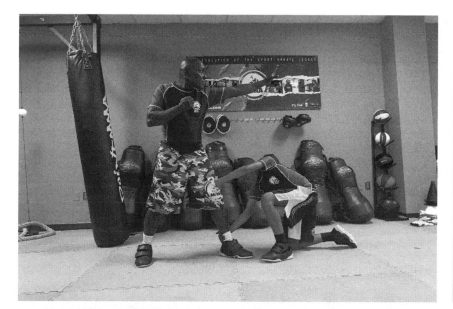
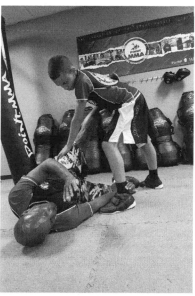

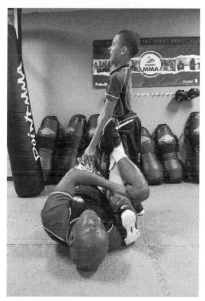
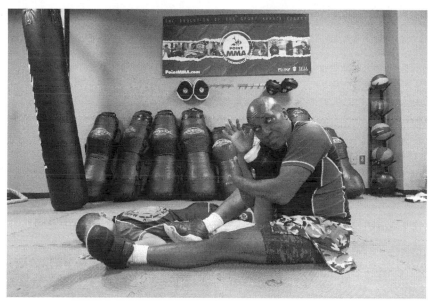

Strive for fluid ground motion. Being able to propel yourself on the ground with a minimum of effort is as important as proper footwork when you're standing, because what's not there, your opponent can't hit. You must be able to move about fluidly by rolling and, at the same time, sweeping with offensive and defensive movements that will position you to win. Believe in your ability and you will be confident on your back. Without confidence, none of the other things will work. There is no secret to developing confidence; it comes through practice and more practice.

Falling Techniques

If you are on the receiving end of a flip, sweep, or takedown, you must be able to maneuver your body into the proper position so you won't get hurt. Be sure your practice sessions include this training.

Backward Fall

Stand with your hands at your sides. Squat down, tuck your chin into your chest, and roll onto your shoulders. As you come out of the tuck position onto your back, slap the mat with your arms extended 45 degrees from your sides, and exhale simultaneously. The key to successful execution is keeping your chin tucked and slapping the mat to break your fall.

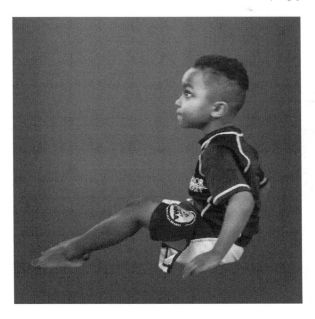 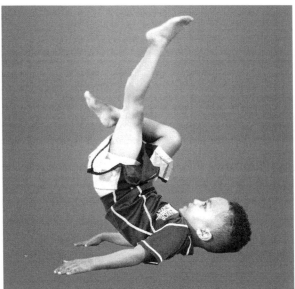

Forward Shoulder Roll

Step forward with your right foot. Using your left arm for support while turning your head to the left, roll across your right arm, across your back, and land on your left arm. Again, it is key to tuck your chin as you go into your roll and to slap the mat and exhale simultaneously to break your fall.

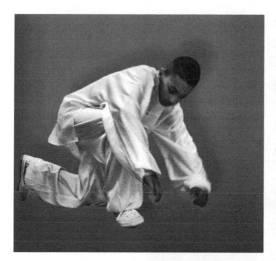
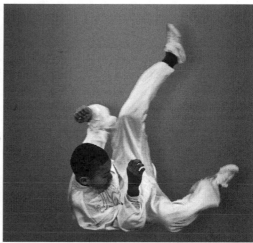

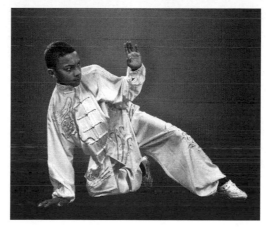

Backward Shoulder Roll

Step back with your left foot and squat down. Keep your knees close to your chest and your chin tucked as you roll over your right shoulder. Avoid hitting your head by using your left hand to guide you.

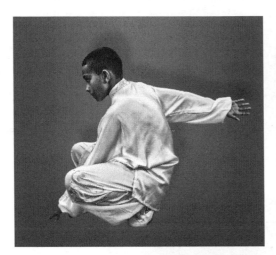
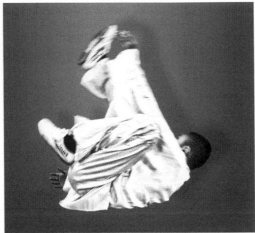
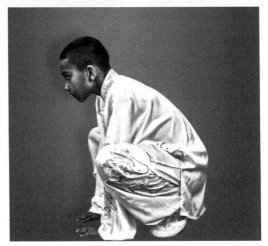

Coordination Drills

These drills develop the necessary attributes to be a spontaneous, natural fighter, one who responds by instinct without forethought. Have you ever watched people dancing who seemed to have two left feet? They stumble and trip over themselves with no rhythm to their movements. To be able to flow with your opponent's tempo, you must first have developed your own rhythm. Once you are comfortable with yourself, you will be much more at ease adapting to your different opponents' rhythms. Mastering coordination drills will give you this edge.

Eyes on Target Drill

Start from the standing on-guard stance and have a partner circle you as you follow, focusing your lead palm on your partner's centerline. As he or she circles, follow with your body and eyes, never letting your partner get inside your hand or behind it. If you are circling to the right, your left hand and leg are in the lead; when circling to the left, your right hand and leg are in the lead. From this posture you can effectively prevent a person from getting inside your body or behind you to attack.

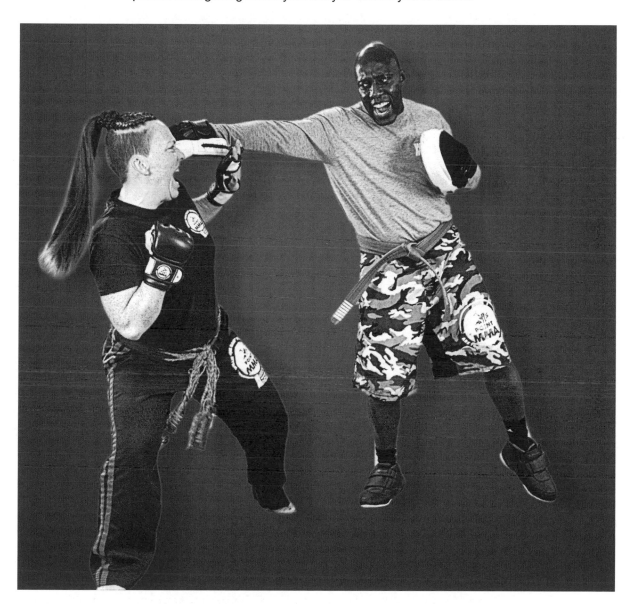

Hand and Foot Drill

Start from the ground and kick your right leg in a cross kick to your partner's right knee. Turn around and execute a left leg round kick. Follow up with a right leg back kick to the body. Stand up and bring your left knee up. Follow with a right elbow strike to the temple. The purpose of this drill is to be able to fluidly move from the ground to a standing position while executing effective techniques.

Hand and foot coordination is key in ground fighting, because your hands might become your legs as you attack or vice versa. Remember, when ground fighting, your hands and feet must work as one.

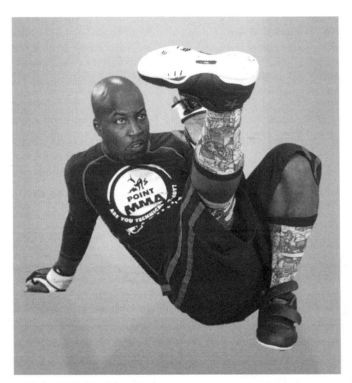

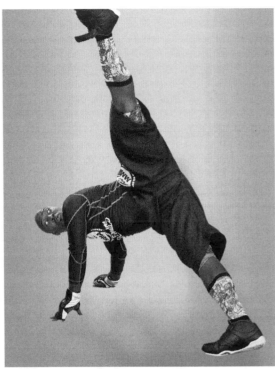

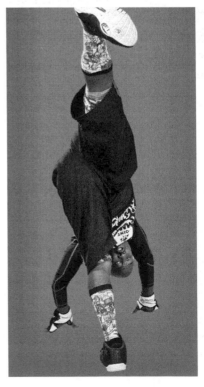

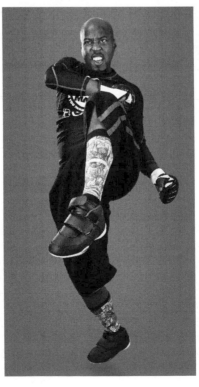

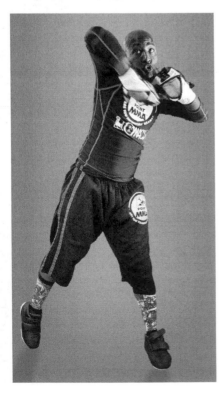

Top and Bottom Grappling

Top and bottom grappling is fighting in a range founded on the premise that you will be at a distinct advantage if you get intimate with your opponent. You can grapple standing up or on the ground. From the grappling range, you can counter your opponent's moves using sensitivity—a key factor in countering. For every effective offensive technique, there is an equally or more effective counter, which you can discover only after you have found harmony of physical motion, not thinking. In combat there is no time to think, everything must be automatic. Thinking is planning, and you must do it beforehand.

There are two ways to fight from the ground. One is striking your opponent, followed by choking and locking him or her into submission. You execute the other by grabbing and holding clothing and flesh to apply an effective choke or joint immobilization. You would commonly use these approaches while standing up as well, which is the sum total of top and bottom defense.

The physical applications of top and bottom grappling are simple, direct, and effective techniques that you can learn in a short time, but to comprehend and internalize these techniques takes years of practice. It is believed that a highly skilled practitioner should be able to destroy and reconstruct in any arena—physical, mental, or spiritual. Used effectively, top and bottom grappling will enhance your foundation. If it's not working for you, it's not the art that's ineffective but your use of it. You must add your personal expression. Store the things that aren't useful for you now and take what is working and use it.

You can best accomplish this through understanding the universal principles and concepts. If you learn only the techniques, you become mechanical; if you understand the principles, you have an arsenal of techniques that are creative and automatic. Couple this with confidence, a belief in your ability, and a commitment to succeed with the skills at hand and you have a formula for success. Regardless of how many grappling techniques you learn, if you never get on the mat and learn how to go with the flow to come out on top with an effective grappling technique, you will be lost in combat.

Keep in mind that it doesn't matter how good you are in grappling. Your first choice is to prevent the confrontation; second, stop the fight as quickly as possible; and third, if a fight is inevitable, fight to win. Also, don't imitate your opponent's moves, but respond to them, because nine times out of ten, your opponent has mastered the moves he or she is executing, and you will end up being the victim. Instead, you need to counter your opponent's techniques with effective moves of your own.

If you do find yourself in a street fight, be prepared to hit the concrete, which may be covered with rocks, broken glass, vomit, or animal waste. Your fighting area may be limited by a building, stairs, cars, or fences. Although years ago, once the hand-to-hand combat was over, the fight was finished, today most opponents on the street are armed with weapons, varying in shape, size, and use. So it's not enough to concentrate on grappling as taught in martial arts classes—you'd better be aware of your opponent pulling out a weapon and adding that to your encounter. Also, don't forget that your opponent usually has friends nearby who will gang up on you and maybe try to stomp your head into the ground. Street fighting gets ugly.

Jab Elbow Combination

Your opponent attacks you with a jab to the face. You counter with a parry palm block and then use your other arm to execute an elbow strike to the side of your opponent's head. Using the same hand, grab the back of his or her neck and slam your rear knee into the inner thigh as you lock your hand around the neck. Place your forearm on the Adam's apple and bring the head into your belly button. As you sink in your abdominal muscles, lean forward and pull your forearm up to the ceiling. Finish by using your left hand to support your right hand as you cut off your opponent's wind, forcing him or her to submit.

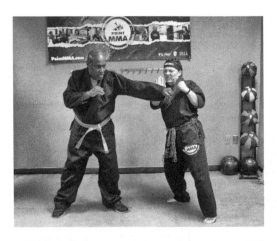
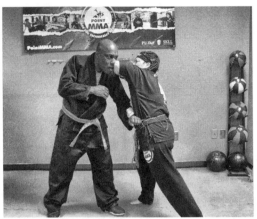
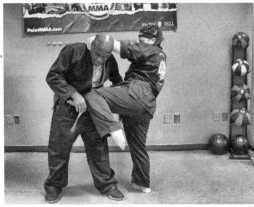
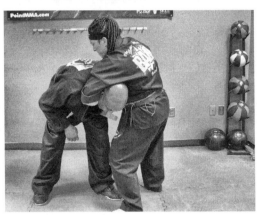
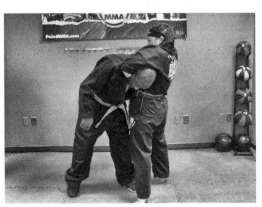

Knee Check Defense

As your opponent rushes forward and forces you to fall over backward, tuck your chin and grab the shoulder or head, lean to the side, and place your knee across the abdomen. Place your free leg outside your opponent's leg, creating a gap between your bodies. Then twist him or her over in a scissors motion with your legs, so your opponent is on his or her back and you're on top in a mount position. From here you should have no trouble executing a choke hold or arm bar.

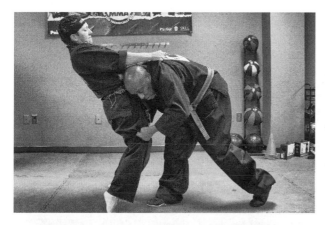
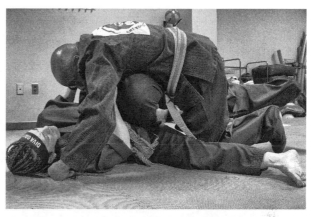
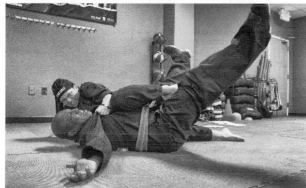
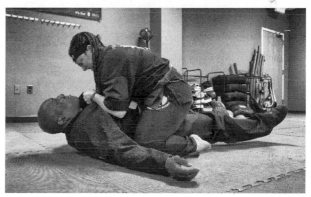

Sparring Tactics

When you go into a fight to win, it is imperative that you employ a method of disposing and maneuvering forces in combat to your advantage. If you just flail about wildly, you will lose in short order. It is, therefore, essential that you understand why you are doing what you're doing, both the advantages and the disadvantages. It isn't enough to know what the basics are; you have to know why each is important and how to use it to win.

Centerline: Draw an imaginary line from the top of your head; through your nose, mouth, and chin; down your breastbone; and across your navel. This is called your centerline, and you must protect it at all times. It is a vulnerable area of the human body, and you can inflict much damage to internal organs along the centerline. Therefore, when fighting, focus all attacks to your opponent's centerline.

At the same time, keep your fists and arms up to block, so your opponent can't get to your centerline. Remember to angle your centerline and use all your body parts as weapons—hands, arms, feet, and legs.

Straight line: The shortest distance between two points is a straight line. That said, it makes sense to hit your opponent with your lead arm or leg. Executing a spinning kick off the back leg may give your opponent the needed moment to move on you. Also, you will gain speed and power when you attack your opponent with a straight-line technique.

Faking: Fake a move or technique to cause your opponent to do what you want him or her to do. Watch how your opponent reacts, taking advantage of the momentary confusion. See if you can fake your opponent into throwing a technique. Use your hips, body, shoulder, hand, leg, or foot to destroy your opponent's timing and scare him or her into moving. Then take advantage of the loss of control and execute.

Bridging the gap: It is important to judge accurately how far away from your opponent you are. Often in a fight, you will see the two fighters touch gloves before they begin. This helps them gauge the distance they will need to cover. Obviously, if you are too far away from your opponent, you will be kicking or punching air. So, you must find a way to bridge the gap while not leaving yourself open. Stay constantly on the move, accentuating your footwork. Use hyperextensions (to extend so the angle of bones in a joint is greater than normal) and faking. You must get in to score and out to keep from getting hit.

Timing: If you are sparring in a tournament, it is always a good idea to score as quickly as you can, before your opponent can move or identify your technique. If you are in a street fight, you may want to wait and see what your opponent is going to throw at you; then counter, being mindful not to overreach. Sometimes good footwork and patience on your part will tire your opponent and leave you an opening for a well-executed technique. Timing is everything.

Constant forward pressure: Use constant mental, aggressive pressure to control your opponent. Even if you are scared to death, don't let it show. In fact, do exactly the reverse. Act extremely confident, aggressive, and not the least bit threatened. Project an inner calmness, even if you don't feel it. Deliver forward techniques to keep your opponent on the defensive. At all times, keep your focus on your goal, which is slipping your opponent's moves.

Mobility: The ability to stay mobile in a fight can save your life. You can't hit a target that's not there, and practice makes perfect in the art of mobility. Using music when you practice will help your rhythm. In a fight, move away only to regroup, and slip in to stay in striking range. Strike, defend, and fake while in motion. Side stepping, back stepping, triangular stepping, circular stepping, and creeping are all effective drills.

Independent movements: These are what you will achieve once you have a strong foundation in basic punching, kicking, stances, footwork, and so on. Too many times I watch a student go into a fight, and start with a kick, pause, then throw a punch, and pause again. To be effective, you must use clean, clear, well-placed techniques in a series that your opponent cannot predetermine. The moves must come to you naturally, but if a judge is watching, there must be no question about which technique you are using. It is only by knowing each move perfectly that you will be able to connect them into a series of effective techniques, and it is only when you can bring a series into the fight that you have found your independent movement. So, respond to whatever your opponent gives you, as with dancing. Stay in harmony with your opponent, and let your body respond as it feels appropriate at the moment.

Bullet speed: Explode into your opponent before he or she can defend. Erupt into your leading offensive and defensive techniques. Push off to gain maximum speed and penetration with your opening techniques, and stay on the move without stopping, no matter what.

Target focus: Guide and direct your attacks to a particular target and stay focused. Wherever your opponent moves, you move and hit, like glue. In defending yourself, however, don't reach—just protect.

Simple technique: Pick three to five techniques that work well for you and master them, avoiding difficult techniques. If you want to win a fight, it's better to rely on the basics and stay away from fancy, show-off techniques. They may look good when you practice them for your friends, but in a fight, while you're trying to pull them off, you may give your opponent the opportunity he or she needs to get in a good punch or kick.

Motion: Staying in motion is a valuable asset. However, don't appear to be running from your opponent. Attack with the weapon closest to the target and use direct angles for attack and defense.

Relaxation: Learning how to relax your body in a fight will take practice. The benefits are that you will conserve your energy and increase your endurance. Relaxing with each offensive technique will increase your delivery speed, and being able to relax your body when defending yourself will enable you to gain control, absorb the blow, and redirect it.

Angles of attack: Although the shortest distance between two points is a straight line, your opponent also knows that and expects this strategy. Therefore, be adept at executing angle to straight-line techniques. Triangular movements will confuse your opponent and possibly give you that split second of opportunity you are waiting for to get a direct hit. It is important that you avoid going toward your opponent's weapons; instead, you must go to the outside and behind that limb. Stay loose so that regardless of which way you move, based on your reaction to your opponent, you must be able to bob and weave or even duck out of striking range. Remember that your body will follow your feet and you can throw your opponent off by going in first one direction and then quickly changing to another. When you're going in for the kill, don't allow your angles to carry you inside toward your opponent's weapons or limbs, which could be dangerous if your defensive skills are weak.

Broken rhythm: Don't get lost in the rhythm of punch, block, kick, block, and so on. Mix the targets and strike your opponent in low, middle, and high ranges. Don't be predictable but be able to change from one rhythm to another at will. Master faking and attacking as well as changing your attitude from aggressive to passive and back to aggressive. Switch your line of attack from inside to outside and back again. Become a master at doing the unexpected. Again, you can't hit a target that's not there.

Sparring Drills

Martial arts were created as a means of self-defense, primarily without weapons. Therefore, every martial arts system has sparring at its core. Sparring allows you to take the basic techniques that you've learned and apply them to controlled fighting situations. You'll get to see how you react under pressure. It is at this stage that I find many students are afraid. They don't want to get hit, and they don't want to do what it takes to learn to counter and defend themselves. There are no shortcuts here. If sparring is the core of martial arts, you must come to terms with it before you can move on and grow in other areas. The following drills will enhance your sparring in combat and competition.

A good workout is several three-minute repetitions of each drill. If that is too intense to begin with, start with one-minute repetitions and work your way up to several three-minute rounds.

Shadow Sparring

Shadow sparring is a form of shadow boxing, which you should do in front of a mirror by watching your shadow or reflection. All you have to do is throw kicks, punches, elbows, knees, and footwork with a free-flowing manner. It also enhances your motion to do this drill to music. By fighting in front of a mirror or watching your shadow on a wall, you can see what your technique looks like. Do a practice repetition and see what you need to correct. However, when you are ready to work out, just let everything flow unconsciously.

Focus Sparring

In this drill you need a partner to hold your target (bag, blocking pad, etc.) and feed you the surface of that target. You need to be able to strike the target with a one, two, three punching combination. It is important that your partner keep the focus glove up in the guard position without showing you the surface until he or she is ready for you to strike it. Each of you must do this drill in a real sparring mood for it to work. Music enhances your rhythm when working this drill. Focus sparring works equally well with kicking, but you will need a handheld kicking shield.

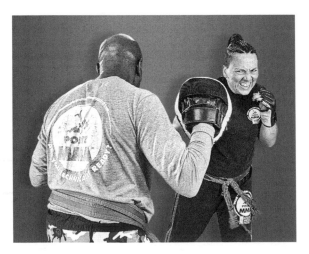

Heavy Bag

Working out with a heavy bag is a great drill to develop a feel for hitting a live opponent. It gives you some idea of the force and speed you will need as opposed to practicing focus sparring. In this drill you freely throw kicks, punches, elbows, and knee strikes at the heavy bag. Again, music plays a good part in helping you develop rhythm. With practice you will be hitting or kicking the bag so hard that it swings back at you, helping you develop a defensive response. It's not a live opponent, but if it swings back and hits you, you'll quickly learn the value of getting out of the way!

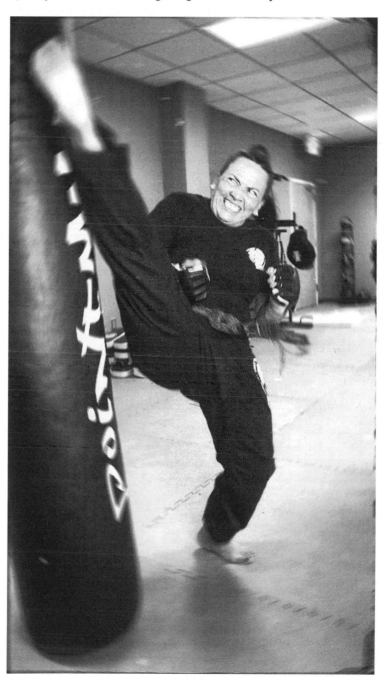

Wing Chun Dummy

One important piece of equipment you can train on to develop trapping, pairing, and centerline defense moves is a wooden wing chun dummy. Practice this drill with free-flowing offensive and defensive moves off the dummy, and make sure you either block with both hands at once or block and strike. It is also important that you block and roll so that some part of your arm is always contacting the dummy. In other words, as long as you are touching the dummy (your pretend opponent), you are in control of the situation or able to counter your opponent's moves. If you break contact, you lose your edge of control.

Rhythm Drill

Work the rhythm drill with a live partner in much the same way as working out with the dummy. Your partner throws a punch and you block; you throw a punch and your partner blocks. There are several combinations, both punching and kicking, that you can use in a two-person rhythm drill, and music is always an aid to timing.

Point Sparring

Point sparring has produced many great kick boxers because it allows you to learn to execute techniques in a controlled manner to any part of your opponent's body. In sport karate, you're only allowed to execute light- or medium-contact techniques to the head-gear, chest, abdominal region, and ribs. Full sparring equipment is mandatory.

Submission Sparring

Submission sparring is not limited to punching, kicking, and sweeps. Today you can add trapping, grappling, and throwing to these techniques. Each time you are successful in executing one of these techniques against your opponent, you get a point. If you apply a submission hold and the victim taps out, you get the point. Always practice this drill on mats and wear personal equipment, including head gear, mouthpiece, chest protector, groin cup (men), shin guards, hand guards, and foot guards. The two people involved directly control the intensity of this drill, because how hard you deliver a blow will determine how hard your opponent counters it. When you are in the heat of this drill, remember to tap out at the slightest inkling of pain. Because your adrenaline is so high, you may be in more danger of injury than you realize.

Circle Sparring

This is one of my favorite drills because it encourages you to be aware of your surroundings. Three to six people form a circle around one person. Then, one by one, they attack the person in the center. The rhythm of this drill is for the person being attacked to have no breaks—no time to think, just respond. An advanced stage of this drill is for everyone to attack the person in the center at the same time, but I wouldn't suggest this until you are a black belt.

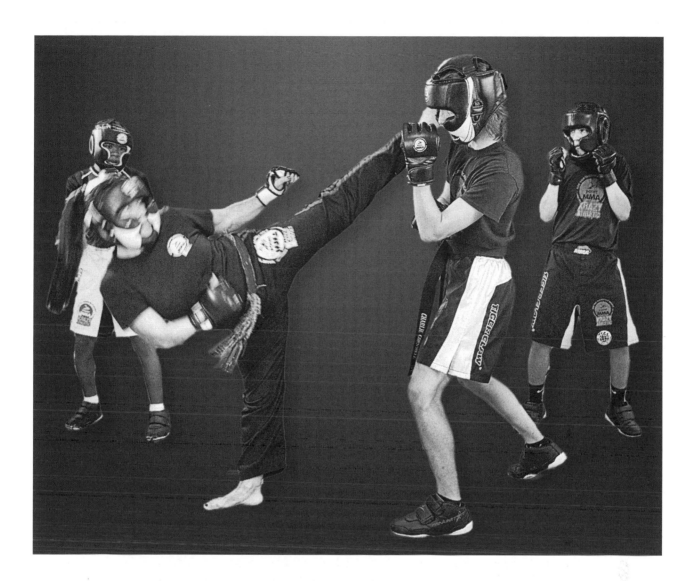

Steps to Winning

Although the steps to becoming a great fighter speak in words directed to people studying martial arts, you can apply them to any pursuit, be it a sport, a profession, or your life. They are words of wisdom that have withstood the test of time. If you approach life with these tools in your toolbox, you will be well prepared to meet life's challenges and come out a winner.

Take your time. A key factor in freestyle sparring or any type of fighting is taking your time—not searching for immediate gratification as our society teaches us. For example, you might try a new combination that doesn't give you the immediate results you want, but by being patient and working repetitions, you will find a successful way to use it.

Use good timing. Timing involves a decision to execute a technique without hesitation when the moment is right. Being too fast or too slow will get you in trouble.

By being there at the right time, you will produce effective results. Life teaches us that when preparation meets opportunity, it far outweighs any amount of talent.

Develop your footwork. Footwork is essential in fighting, and getting from point A to point B as fast as possible is crucial, so you must master your footwork pattern. Work your system over and over, and don't forget to use visualization in this learning process. A little extra time here while you establish a solid base can make all the difference in getting out of the way of something coming at you. After all, it's going to be hard to strike your opponent if you're already lying on the mat!

Learn from confrontation. For you to grow past your fears, you must confront them head on. Everything in martial arts comes down to confrontation or facing up to something. Sooner or later, even wearing sparring equipment, you're going to be on the receiving end of a blow or two. You may get the wind knocked out of you or a split lip, and I'm talking about in the classroom. To become a fighter, it is necessary for you to get past being angry, to get past the pain, and to evaluate what happened from the technical side. Face your weak areas and build them up. In other words, learn from your mistakes.

Be aware of your surroundings. When sparring, you must be aware of not only your range of combat but also your opponent's. Remain alert to your opponent's actions while not freezing from tension. You will be amazed at what you can see when you expand your space to include your opponent.

Practice being universal. In sparring it is easy to develop favorite techniques and use them all the time. Beware! Certain things will work only on certain people. You must become a universal fighter, adapting and moving in rhythm to your opponent's movements. Apply this in techniques, footwork, target, and thinking. Use no patterns at all, just action and response.

Stay conscious of yourself at all times. In many sparring matches there is an attacker and a counterattacker. When executing a technique as the attacker, you must be totally committed on the physical level. Mentally and emotionally you must remain loose and free to respond to whatever takes place. When you can flow as one with the universe, you will have learned a valuable lesson.

Responding under pressure. Freestyle sparring is a great way to develop your ability to respond under pressure. Frequently in sparring sessions, a student's mind locks when the opponent is constantly throwing techniques or when he or she gets tired or scared. At this point you should be responding to what is in front of you, not analyzing your thoughts and emotions. This analyzing and thinking is done before you ever get in a combative situation. The key is to stay conscious of what is going on at all times, to be fast on your feet, and, above all, to be able to respond under pressure.

Control your emotions. If you want to win your match, controlling your emotions is essential. If you are being hit more often than your opponent, anger may flare up along with feelings of frustration, shame, and loss of control. When your emotions take over, your ability to execute techniques gets worse because you are not in control of the match any more. To be in control, you need to embrace these emotions and direct them toward winning.

Maintain control even when your opponent tries to trick you. It's simply an attitude of mind over matter. You have to believe in yourself from the inside, so your attitude and spirit become strong. This is the perfect time to showcase your champion attitude. Now your techniques will match your spirit, appearing well placed and strong. The moment your opponent loses control, you are there smiling, ready to react to the uncontrolled movements.

Be yourself. When practicing, it is important not to become a clone of the other students or your instructor but to continually develop your individual expression—physically, mentally, and spiritually—by combining the proper principles, techniques, and approaches. In the martial arts, the degree to which you can express a particular action, principle, or approach to someone else parallels your ability to execute it. Be yourself!

> Continually develop your individual expression—physically, mentally, and spiritually—by combining the proper principles, techniques, and approaches.

Follow your instincts. Being true to your nature is key to flowing in harmony with the universe. An aikido expert calls it qi. Others call it your sixth sense. This is expressed by being in tune with yourself consciously and unconsciously. You must not try to feel or receive, but simply *be* the situation. Act on your gut feelings, first an action, then a response, an action and a response, back and forth. Focus on your successes. Follow your instincts and go with the flow.

Many people study martial arts because they want to develop their fighting skills, then have a chance to go one-on-one with other martial artists. It seems more refined and socially acceptable to them than going outside and picking a fight with someone on the street. Of course you don't get the same possible dire consequences, because there is always a measure of controlled fighting in the ring. However, the ultimate measure of martial artists is not their ability to fight but their capacity to avoid fighting in the first place. Competitive sparring at tournaments is simply a proving ground to experience your physical, mental, and spiritual prowess on the battlefield. It is where you gain control of the emotions you feel under stress or an out-of-control situation. The reward is to develop your self-confidence to such a high level that you know you can protect yourself and win, and fighting isn't necessary at all.

However, if the situation arises that you must engage in combat, allow your attributes to accelerate your techniques in a natural manner that's appropriate to your opponent's attack. For example, if your opponent pulls you forward, push yourself forward into him or her, or if your opponent pushes you, grab anywhere you can and pull him or her into you. You are now in tune with the situation and responding with a natural give-and-take. This is the ultimate manifestation of universal sparring.

The Road to Success

6

Once you become aware of the truth, ignorance isn't an option

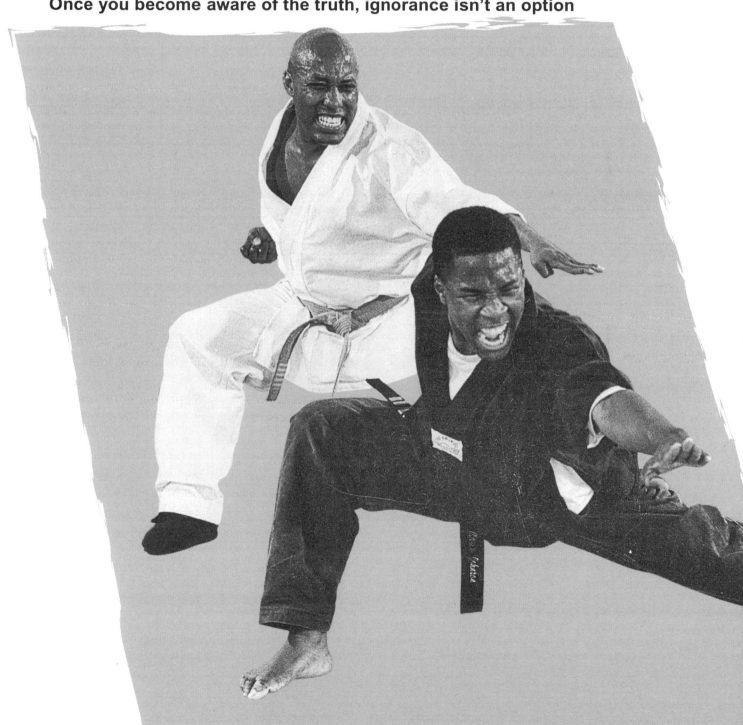

People spend thousands of dollars for dream martial arts programs—programs that develop self-confidence, discipline, enthusiasm, respect, and a spirit of teamwork while honing their individual skills. These people can also choose to join a health club or a sports team to get many of the same benefits. The difference for serious martial artists is that sooner or later they face the fact that this is not just a way to get physically in shape, a fun activity that reduces stress, or a chance to play a team sport. Those who adopt martial arts as a way of life discover that the road to their success is an inside job.

The Choice Is Yours

What you do and how hard you push yourself when you're alone is what helps you stand out from the crowd. The Universal Creator created us as unique individuals with no guilt, free to express ourselves. It's always easy to start something new. The challenge is to stay dedicated and see it through to a successful conclusion.

> What you do and how hard you push
> is what sets you apart from the masses.

Today's students enter their dream martial arts program, and everything they hoped for is coming true. They are in the best physical shape of their lives; their levels of self-confidence, discipline, enthusiasm, and awareness are at an all-time high. As a side benefit, these attributes flow into other areas of their lives, and they reap extraordinary successes outside the school. Many students report improved personal and family relationships as well as outstanding yearly performance evaluations at work. Sometimes these successes spell job promotion and relocation hundreds of miles from their school.

What next? thinks the student. *How do I keep up my training? I don't want to start over in another school or discipline.* (Ranks don't transfer from one martial arts school to another. If you go to a second school to study, you would again be a beginning, white belt student.) *How can I keep from falling behind? Should I stop?*

The truth is, students need ask none of these questions, because the ultimate goal in martial arts training is to be self-motivated. A martial arts school that embraces martial arts as a way of life will work with you, helping you plan a workout schedule that keeps you in shape and a curriculum for your progress. You should be able to work out anywhere in the world. The dojo is inside you, whether you realize it or not. All these people, places, and things outside yourself are merely tools that bring you closer to this truth, but you will have to make the commitment to yourself to do it. Self-motivation is what separates the winners from the losers, a dedicated martial artist from a weekend warrior. Suppose the time comes when you have to dig deep to find the motivation to continue something you've started or to do what has helped you succeed in the past. Everyone I know has to cross this hurdle sometime. Most people run from these challenges by switching to something else and make up excuses for why they aren't succeeding.

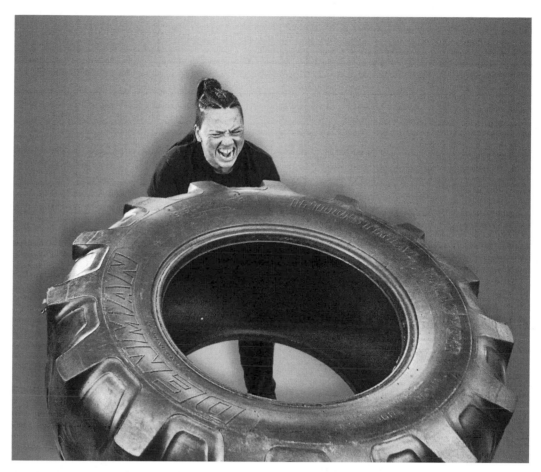

Sometimes you have to dig deep to find extra strength and self-motivation.

There is a secret to help you out of your slump. It is to go with the flow and stick to the basics, even when they're no longer fun. Eventually all the bad moments will flow into good—it's a law of nature. The hardest thing about trying to help students understand this experience is that there is no single reason this happens. It's one of those things in life that just is. It's like having a head cold. You don't know where it came from or how long you will have it, but you do know that eventually it will go away if you take care of yourself. The same rule applies here.

Many people look at my life and say they are sorry for the things I have had to go through. They wish I hadn't had so many hard times, but I tell everyone that I'm glad I went through what I did. I learned many valuable lessons, including how to motivate myself and how to keep my attitude positive.

Even when I was homeless, I carried my martial arts portfolio, weapons, and writing plans with me. I continued to work out every day, wherever I was, and I never stopped dreaming of the things that are manifesting in my life today. This is true self-motivation, to keep going when there's no support, no rewards, no pats on the back, just self-satisfaction in knowing you're doing the right thing for the right reasons.

Establishing a Training Plan

If you are traveling or have to move, be cautious about training in another martial arts school. It could limit you if it doesn't encourage individual self-expression. At my school I gear what I teach to enhance each individual's well-being. I encourage students to try many things and find the techniques that work for them.

> Always choose a school
> that encourages your self-expression.

If you decide to change schools for whatever reason, I feel that what you have achieved should be recognizable by the example you set and how you display your ability. I don't believe in telling someone you have a black belt or any belt to get special treatment, and even when they find out, you should humbly admit it. I would decline any special treatment, because it usually brings bad feelings among students who have been training at the school longer than you have. On the other hand, I think the school should allow you to express or work on what you have achieved and support you in combining your foundation with the new techniques you're learning, as long as you do it respectfully and in a manner that doesn't create conflict.

My experience is that if you honestly do this, the instructor will support you in this self-expression and allow you to do what comes naturally for you. If not, you need to move on, because you should have an environment that lets you express yourself to your fullest potential.

If you opt for home training, you are the instructor and coach. This is what self-motivation is about. You have to guide yourself in becoming the best martial artist you can be.

The reality is that you should be doing these things every day to complement your classes: exercising, something aerobic such as running or jumping rope, practicing punches and kicks, working through a form. Then if you find yourself traveling on a business trip, away on vacation, or thrust into a move, you already have established a home workout routine. You simply continue as you have been.

When you train at home, you can practice techniques from any style, system, or concept. There are no limits, because in this situation, individual expression is the goal. For students who are beginning martial arts training, say in their first year, it is important that whatever they practice be an extension of what they learn in the classroom. Wait until you have participated in one art form for a few years and have your foundation firmly in place before studying something else.

Building Strength and Endurance

Being in good physical shape is where it begins. Until you have exercised and conditioned your muscles, they won't be able to perform. So, let's start with getting your muscles ready. Most people say that they push themselves hardest when they are following exercises with an instructor or coach. Therefore, when you aren't in class working out, I suggest that you do at least as much as you would in a class and add another 10 percent.

Jumping rope, running, and jumping jacks will build cardiovascular endurance. Try sit-ups, crunches, and leg lifts to build your abdominal muscles so you can take a punch, and kicks and punches to strengthen your legs and arms for fighting. Don't forget push-ups for building upper-body strength. It would be reasonable to start with one repetition of fifty of each exercise as a first-year student and work your way up to several hundred of each. Joining a health club and working out on their equipment is another option.

Music is a great tool, and I always use it to accompany my workouts. Once again, self-motivation is the key and music is my motivator. I use all kinds—hip-hop, rock, rhythm and blues, pop, techno, new age, classical, and so on. It depends on the mood I'm in and the emotions I'm trying to bring forth.

Increasing Your Flexibility

Stretching is another important aspect in martial arts development. Whichever concept of martial arts you study has its own stretching and warm-up routines. Remember to put some of these at the beginning and end of your workout.

Upper-Torso Stretch

One of my favorites, involves an upper-torso stretch that targets the side and back muscles, the hamstrings, and the calf muscles. Begin by standing in a relaxed position with your feet at least shoulder-width apart and your hands at your sides. Bring your arms overhead, interlock your fingers (a), and stretch your arms down between your legs, trying to touch the floor (b). Then bring your arms back overhead and return them to your sides. Repeat this two more times. However, on the third time, when your hands are overhead, instead of dropping them to your sides, turn your body slightly to the right and make three rotations from overhead to the floor (c, d); then turn to the left and make three rotations. Finish by bringing your hands in front of you at chest height, then down to the floor in front of you, then to the right (e), the left, and once more in front. Bring your hands overhead one last time and return them to your sides. As you go through the positions, hold each one for three to five seconds or longer. Do at least three of these for a proper warm-up.

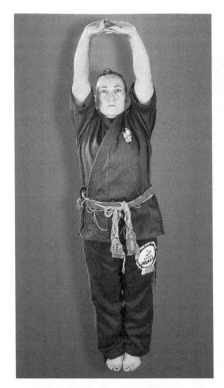

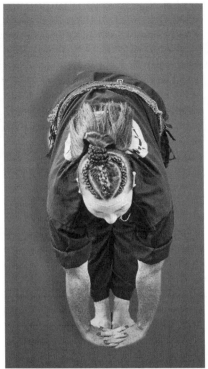

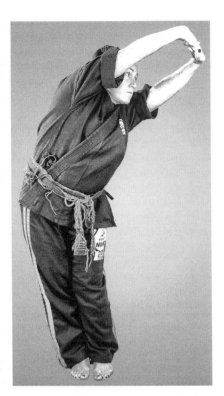

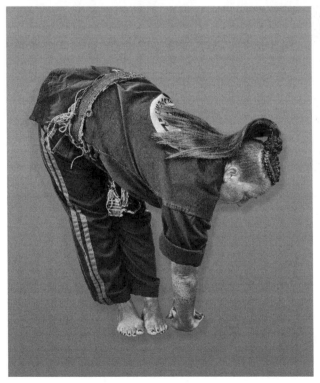

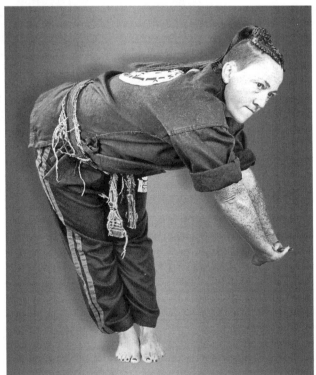

Hamstring Stretch

You can develop and stretch the hamstring and calf muscles by standing with your feet no wider than your shoulders and your hands at your sides. Shift your weight to one leg and extend your other foot to the front with your weight on your heel, toes pointed upward. Bend your elbow on the same side as your extended foot and try to touch your elbow to your toes. Hold this stretch for three to five seconds. Repeat this stretch with your other foot and elbow. Six to eight repetitions are my normal warm-up.

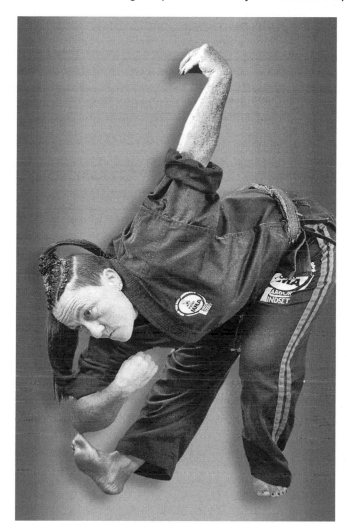

Drop-Stance Stretch

The drop-stance stretch benefits the thigh, hamstring, and calf muscles. Start with your legs a minimum of shoulder-width apart and your hands on your hips. Drop to your right side by bending your right knee, extending your left leg and keeping both feet flat on the floor. Turn your upper torso slightly to the left and inside your extended left leg. Come up and drop to your left, extending your right leg and bending your body to the right and slightly inside your extended right leg. Again, six to eight repetitions will adequately warm and stretch these muscles.

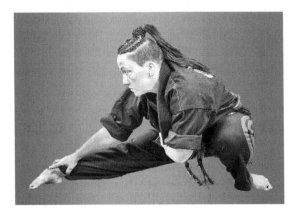

Circular Stretches

Wrists, ankles, and knees will benefit from circular rotations of eight to ten turns to the left and another eight to ten to the right. You can rotate your shoulders and arms forward and backward eight to ten times each. Turn your head left and right, up and down, and from side to side in a semicircular motion at least ten times each.

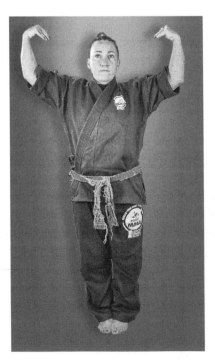

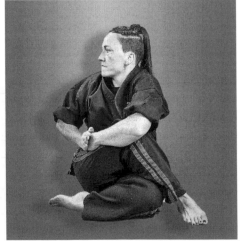

Hip Stretch

You can stretch hip muscles by sitting on the floor and bringing one foot to the inside of your thigh. Take your other leg to the opposite side, crossing your bent leg, and placing your foot flat on the floor. Holding your knee with your stationary arms, turn your chest toward your knee, hold, and feel the stretch. Then do the other side. Be sure to hold each stretch for at least ten seconds, alternating from side to side with five repetitions each.

Practicing Basic Techniques

Basic movements are every martial artist's foundation. When you are in a martial arts school, request a copy of your school curriculum—all professional schools should have a curriculum for each level. Armed with this information, you can decide exactly what you want to work on, vary your routines, and be sure you stay on track by learning exactly what you will be tested on.

Some basics include punching, blocking, footwork, and kicks. I recommend focusing on one area of basics each week. Then you can perfect this area before moving to the next. The last week of each month, combine the basic moves you have been working on. If your school or instructor doesn't have a written curriculum to give you, take notes on everything you learn in class, at seminars, and on video. Ask your instructor if you can film training techniques.

Visualizing Advanced Techniques

Going beyond the basics to work on your forms, weapons routines, self-defense, and fighting is challenging. If you have training equipment at home, such as speed bags and heavy bags, these will help tremendously. If not, I suggest that when you work on a form or weapon routine, you should be able to practice it in a small area. Change your footwork and arm extensions to accommodate the space available. Visualize your movements while you're lying in bed or meditating. With your eyes closed, picture every punch, block, and kick. Break them into the finest detail. Also, if possible, tape your form and watch it repeatedly. Some people find that writing each movement of a form, detail by detail, helps them remember the different parts. Find a way that works for you, then spend at least ten minutes a day, every day, visualizing. It works!

> Visualization is one of the most powerful techniques you can add to your training.

When learning self-defense techniques and fighting, use the same visualization techniques already mentioned. Pretend you have an opponent. There is a strong connection between what you put in your mind and what your body can give out.

Home training is not better than being in a school, and being in a school is not better than home training. They complement each other. Now that you know this, you should have no problem or excuse about continuing your training regardless of the situation.

Practicing Good Nutrition

Good nutrition and eating habits were not part of my lifestyle. I had no idea that the better you eat, the better you feel. Coming up poor, we ate whatever we had and didn't pay any attention to how healthful it was for us. After my mom died, I kept eating those fried, greasy foods; red meat; pork; sodas; and desserts loaded with sugar. I remember when I was training with Master Brown, who is a vegetarian, he and his wife had me over for dinner and told me how these foods affected my body, but at the time I wasn't the least bit interested in good eating habits. Either I didn't eat anything, or I overindulged and ate everything I could get my hands on.

I got my first taste of eating balanced meals three times a day while I was incarcerated, and I met some inmates who turned me on to eating healthful meals and reading books on nutrition. When I got out, I hung around martial artists who practiced good eating habits, and I read what people like Tony Robbins and Bruce Lee had to say about eating right to stay in shape. I began subtracting meat and soda from my diet. Then I began taking vitamins every day, drinking a glass of fresh-squeezed juice every morning, and eating plenty of fish. Today, I work out and teach martial arts six days a week. I find my body works and feels its best with one full-course, all-natural meal a day, supplemented with fresh-squeezed juices and vitamins. I'm not recommending this diet for you. I am simply sharing what I have found, through trial and error, works best for me. You will need to discover what works for you. For some, it may mean eating three well-balanced meals a day. Others might find that having five small meals or snacks will give them the energy and stamina they need.

> Find a diet that gives your body the right combination of foods at the right time of day, then stick to it.

My newly-discovered good eating habits have carried into what I ask my black belt candidates to adhere to during a testing cycle. Requirements include no red meat or pork, no fried foods, no caffeine or refined sugar, and no eating after 9 p.m. Believe it or not, the students start out being unenthusiastic about the changes in their diets, but at the end of their three-month testing cycle, they are usually amazed at how much energy they have, how well their bodies are operating, and how well they feel.

The downside is that most people go back to their old ways. It's hard, but like everything else, you must think about the consequences of what you are about to put into your mouth and how it will affect you physically, mentally, and spiritually.

Responding the Right Way

Life is a journey that happens while we are making other plans. Its beginning started for each of us the day we were born; the ending is guaranteed. What happens in the seconds, minutes, hours, days, weeks, and years is not always our choice—that's a fact. Where you do have the choice is deciding how you are going to respond in any situation. Please notice that I said respond here, not react. Responding comes from a base of personal control and levelheadedness, regardless of whether you weigh your decision in seconds or years. Reacting, on the other hand, is like a knee-jerk movement to something that happens, an instinctual move with little base other than spur of the moment. Each has its place and time.

Sample Meal Plan

The human body is an amazing vehicle. Although a car runs on gasoline, and all you have to do is fill the gas tank and keep going until you reach empty, animals have a much more delicate balance to keep their engines running efficiently. Knowing what kinds of food will give you energy, endurance, and brain power, and when during each twenty-four-hour period you need to consume them is unique to each individual. The following is a sample meal plan. Experiment with it and get to know your body's needs. I promise that if you take the time to do this, you will begin to recognize the big and little signals all parts of your body send and learn exactly when and what you need to eat or drink to feel your best.

Breakfast

One eight- to twelve-ounce glass of fresh-squeezed fruit juice. Choose one or more of the following: apple, cherry, pineapple, lemon, pear, orange, banana, raspberry, grapefruit, and so on.

One toasted bagel with toppings as desired. Two eight-ounce glasses of water.

Sundays only: Two slices of French toast. Two tablespoons of Log Cabin Lite syrup.

One scrambled egg with Pam or three egg whites. Two eight-ounce glasses of water.

Lunch or Dinner

One eight- to twelve-ounce glass of fruit or vegetable juice, fresh-squeezed. I especially like a combination of apples and carrots with a little fresh ginger root.

Choose one of the following or something similar: six-ounce catfish fillet, shrimp lo mein, tuna fish sandwich, or veggie burger.

Choose two of the following: two to three cups of garden salad with light salad dressing, one cup of broccoli, one half cup of corn, one cup of green beans, two cups of spinach, or eight to sixteen ounces of V-8 or tomato juice.

Three eight-ounce glasses of water.

Snacks

You can eat snacks throughout the day.

One glass of vegetable juice-any combination of vegetables and any size glass.

Fresh fruits as desired: one apple, one banana, one cup grapes, one orange, two cups strawberries, two peaches. It's OK to eat all these fruits in a day as long as you don't exceed the quantity specified.

Unlimited water.

One glass of fruit juice.

No eating after 9 p.m.

For instance, if someone says something to you that provokes your anger, you have a choice to respond or react. If you choose to respond, you may not say anything at the moment but go away to compose yourself, deal with your anger without venting at the person, and, when you are done being angry, you are operating from a position of personal control. You now have the advantage and can go back to say whatever you need to say.

If you react in anger to what someone says or does to you, you are at a serious disadvantage. You will be in a confrontation instigated by someone who is probably in control of themselves, while you are flailing in retaliation with not much chance of getting your needs met.

> Beware of reacting in anger,
> because this puts your opponent in control.

Our ultimate goal is to flow and respond in the proper manner right then and there. Whatever happens should contribute to the lessons you are learning at this time. Everything is connected, producing a chain reaction. When you react to someone, it produces stagnation and the flow stops, but when you respond, it creates a peaceful connection. Within this connection anger, frustration, sadness, humility, and all types of emotions occur, but they are within a circle of peace. I use a circle as an example because what goes around, comes around. Someday you will meet the other side of your reaction or response. Your best choice, then, is to contribute to the flow with peace, love, and happiness.

If you can't respond with peace, because things happen that we haven't thought about, try to stay in a state of nonattachment. In other words, it is inevitable that things will happen throughout your day that are unexpected, and some will probably be challenging, even upsetting. The secret to getting through these situations without coming unglued is to not get personally attached. Simply accept them as little pebbles in life's stream for you to endure for the moment. They won't last forever. Just do the next right thing, knowing that the Universal Creator is ultimately in charge anyway.

Once you can define the difference between responding and reacting, it will be clear that you do have a choice in your behavior. It is my firm belief that if I am going to get the consequences of my actions, then I am going to take responsibility for making my decisions and not give this power away to anyone. That said, the span of your life, from birth to death, is yours to use as you see fit. It is the Universal Creator's gift to you. You didn't ask for it, but it definitely is yours. What you do with your life is up to you, and if you think about it, it is your gift to the Universal Creator.

Your mind is always trying to figure out how, when, and why it should respond in a certain way, but the key is to just be. Through self-examination you will develop an awareness of the pure possibilities available to you and be able to use them the next time. Never dwell on how much success you achieve, and never grow satisfied or complacent. That state of mind brings only sorrow, sadness, and disappointment.

Many of us have been going along from day to day and year to year letting life happen to us. Yes, there have been times we made conscious choices that affected results in our lives. Possibly you decided to go to college to get a degree, which placed you in a career field that you like. Perhaps you sent out job applications to places you wanted to work, then selected a job you thought was right. You married the perfect person to be the mother or father of your children. You bought a house in a neighborhood with good schools for your children. You worshiped in a religious family with values similar to your own. You even studied martial arts so you can defend yourself and stay physically, mentally, and spiritually fit.

However, it's the time between these choices that I'm talking about. That's the time things seem to happen to us. That's life—it's what is happening while we're formulating the next, usually big, plan. I would say it makes up more than half of anyone's life. Therefore, it might be in your best interest to be conscious of how you're spending all this time. For many of you, this may be the first time you stopped to think about what you do when you are between achieving your goals; how you conduct yourself; how other people see you; and what your behaviors, attitudes, principles, values, and morals are.

> Stop and think carefully about how you want to spend
> your time between achieving your goals—
> it's more than half your lifetime.

The truth is that we are free to use our time any way we want, as long as we understand that with this freedom comes responsibility. Never allow other people, places, and things to influence your choice. Only you and the Universal Creator have this right, and nothing should rob you of that. If someone does, which is a common thing, you must be secure enough with yourself and the Universal Creator to stand up and live with the consequences.

At any moment when something happens and you have to choose whether you are going to react or respond, it is better to come from a base of facts rather than feelings, but here is the paradox. At certain times reacting is necessary, and at other times responding is necessary. The moment for deciding is solely based on your inner sensitivity to the situation. You must be so in tune with yourself that you instinctively make the decision that is right for the moment.

I wrote this book as a guide for you to start thinking about these things—who you are and how you want to use this gift your Universal Creator has given you.

I wrote it from my base of experience as a martial artist. Therefore, it may be easy for fellow martial artists to identify with, but I hope you can go beyond the framework within which I chose to develop myself and see the big picture. Reach for the understanding that there's more to life than acting and reacting, more than getting up, going to school or work, coming home, and going to bed. If that's all there is in your life, I think it's time to take another look and make some new choices, or at least different ones.

Martial arts are not just hobbies or sports, except for those people who take classes and forget what they've learned as soon as they walk out the door. A martial artist is someone who adopts the principles that have been passed down from generation to generation as their way of life. It is as much who they are as their gender. They are constantly searching to find balance, to have inner peace and happiness, to be useful to humankind, to leave positive footprints while they are here on earth. The Universal Creator gives us His unconditional love. Should we not love ourselves enough to reach for our highest level of understanding—to give 110 percent and do our best with every opportunity set in our path?

110-Percent Martial Arts Theory

True martial artists, those people who have made a commitment to the martial arts principles, have also made a commitment to themselves and the Universal Creator to reach for their highest level of understanding. We are not satisfied with doing only what is required, even if we do it perfectly. We must always go beyond, seeking to give 110 percent to every opportunity placed in our path.

20 percent gifted real-life ability.

15 percent physical martial arts instruction.

10 percent sport martial arts science, external achievement, and universal respect.

15 percent conscious and unconscious awareness of the inner self, mental toughness, and manifested discipline and respect.

20 percent spiritual development maintained through a daily regime of prayer, meditation, spiritual reading, studying, and discussion.

20 percent universal harmony achieved by working the principles in this book.

10 percent is to just do, be into each second, which influences each minute, hour, day, week, month, and year.

You may want to reread this book now and take stock of where you are with the twelve principles in chapter 2. Take an inventory of your ability level and identify the areas you want to work on today and those things you will save for later. Remember to strive for perfection, realizing that you will never attain it, but through every attempt, you will make progress.

> Remember to strive for perfection,
> realizing that you will never attain it,
> but through every attempt, you will make progress.

Those people who lead a principle-centered life will be criticized and disliked by many, but they should never compromise their standards or character. They shouldn't reveal their sharpness too much either but take everything that happens to them and use it as a form of medicine that helps them refine their character. Through this, your heart and soul become genuine, and you will affect the world positively, bringing about balance among people, places, and things. This is the martial arts way. Don't claim to create it, master it, or be it; just discover it by embracing and working the principles in this book.

> We are neither spokespeople nor interpreters
> of any one way, but strive to be part of all ways
> while recognizing that human beings are messengers
> for a power greater than ourselves.

May peace be with you always!

A seven-time Karate and Kung Fu world champion and two-time All-American champion, **Willie "The BAM" Johnson** is a true hero in the world of martial arts. As the creator of Wushudo Universal Martial Arts, Johnson is known for his dynamic, universal approach to developing physical, mental, and spiritual fitness. He is the co-owner and president of The BAMS Martial Arts Academy with his wife Kimberly Johnson in Laurel, Maryland, open for twenty-five years. In 1991, Johnson made history as America's first nationally ranked Triple Crown martial arts champion. Only three years later, he had the distinction of being the first African-American to be ranked number one in Kung Fu forms and weapons.

In addition to these accomplishments, he has earned fifth- and seventh-degree black belts in Karate and Kung Fu and studied several other arts such as Jujitsu, Thai boxing, boxing, wrestling, Tai Chi and kickboxing. Johnson received the title of Grand Master in 1995 and is a member of the Martial Arts Hall of Fame. He starred as himself on the WMAC Masters television show and the Wesley Snipes *Masters of the Martial Arts* show. He is also the creator of the Predator's Self-Defense Concepts, which teaches all participants how to deal with the deadly predators that stalk individuals within society. In 2000, he was named Kung Fu Instructor of the Year by *Black Belt Magazine*, and appeared on the cover of that magazine in 2018.

A graduate of the Beijing Physical Culture Institute of China, Johnson has nearly thirty years of training in the martial arts. He has appeared in four films, including *Super Fighters* and *Major League II,* sixteen stage plays, eleven television shows, and two videos. He has also had more than thirty articles published in leading martial arts magazines and been featured on the cover of *Karate/Kung Fu Illustrated* and *Martial Arts Training.*

Named Instructor of the Year by the Educational Funding Corporation, Johnson is the founder and national spokesperson for the Stronger Than Drugs Foundation. He is a regional representative of the U.S. Shuai Chiao Association and the Federation of United Martial Artist Crusade Against Crime. In addition to these contributions, he serves as national spokesperson for Champions Against Drugs and grand master of the World Head of Family Sokeship Council. He is a member of the Educational Funding Corporation and the National Professional Association of Martial Artists. Johnson is also the founder and coach of the leading sport karate team known as the Better Attitude Makers, and founder of the Cardio Defense Kickboxing program. Mr. Johnson, his family and his academy participate in an annual food drive, toy drive, and provide blessing bags for the homeless each year among other community service activities. Johnson resides in Columbia, Maryland.

About the Authors

A seven-time Karate and Kung Fu world champion and two-time All-American champion, **Willie "The BAM" Johnson** is a true hero in the world of martial arts. As the creator of Wushudo Universal Martial Arts, Johnson is known for his dynamic, universal approach to developing physical, mental, and spiritual fitness. He is the co-owner and president of The BAMS Martial Arts Academy with his wife Kimberly Johnson in Laurel, Maryland, open for twenty-five years. In 1991, Johnson made history as America's first nationally ranked Triple Crown martial arts champion. Only three years later, he had the distinction of being the first African-American to be ranked number one in Kung Fu forms and weapons.

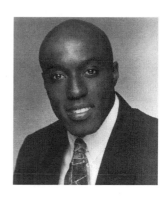

In addition to these accomplishments, he has earned fifth- and seventh-degree black belts in Karate and Kung Fu and studied several other arts such as Jujitsu, Thai boxing, boxing, wrestling, Tai Chi and kickboxing. Johnson received the title of Grand Master in 1995 and is a member of the Martial Arts Hall of Fame. He starred as himself on the WMAC Masters television show and the Wesley Snipes *Masters of the Martial Arts* show. He is also the creator of the Predator's Self-Defense Concepts, which teaches all participants how to deal with the deadly predators that stalk individuals within society. In 2000, he was named Kung Fu Instructor of the Year by *Black Belt Magazine*, and appeared on the cover of that magazine in 2018.

A graduate of the Beijing Physical Culture Institute of China, Johnson has nearly thirty years of training in the martial arts. He has appeared in four films, including *Super Fighters* and *Major League II,* sixteen stage plays, eleven television shows, and two videos. He has also had more than thirty articles published in leading martial arts magazines and been featured on the cover of *Karate/Kung Fu Illustrated* and *Martial Arts Training.*

Named Instructor of the Year by the Educational Funding Corporation, Johnson is the founder and national spokesperson for the Stronger Than Drugs Foundation. He is a regional representative of the U.S. Shuai Chiao Association and the Federation of United Martial Artist Crusade Against Crime. In addition to these contributions, he serves as national spokesperson for Champions Against Drugs and grand master of the World Head of Family Sokeship Council. He is a member of the Educational Funding Corporation and the National Professional Association of Martial Artists. Johnson is also the founder and coach of the leading sport karate team known as the Better Attitude Makers, and founder of the Cardio Defense Kickboxing program. Mr. Johnson, his family and his academy participate in an annual food drive, toy drive, and provide blessing bags for the homeless each year among other community service activities. Johnson resides in Columbia, Maryland.

Nancy Holt Musick, program review coordinator for the American Council on Education, has a lifetime commitment to growing physically, mentally, and spiritually. Musick has earned a first-degree black belt under Johnson and served as a student instructor at the Universal Martial Arts Concepts school. A member of the Special Winning Attitude Team at "The BAMS", she has had more than thirty articles published in leadng martial arts magazines. Musick resides in Centervlle, Virginia and is an avid writer and fitness buff.

BOOKS FROM YMAA

101 REFLECTIONS ON TAI CHI CHUAN
108 INSIGHTS INTO TAI CHI CHUAN
A SUDDEN DAWN: THE EPIC JOURNEY OF BODHIDHARMA
A WOMAN'S QIGONG GUIDE
ADVANCING IN TAE KWON DO
ANALYSIS OF SHAOLIN CHIN NA 2ND ED
ANCIENT CHINESE WEAPONS
THE ART AND SCIENCE OF STAFF FIGHTING
ART OF HOJO UNDO
ARTHRITIS RELIEF, 3D ED.
BACK PAIN RELIEF, 2ND ED.
BAGUAZHANG, 2ND ED.
BRAIN FITNESS
CARDIO KICKBOXING ELITE
CHIN NA IN GROUND FIGHTING
CHINESE FAST WRESTLING
CHINESE FITNESS
CHINESE TUI NA MASSAGE
CHOJUN
COMPLETE MARTIAL ARTIST
COMPREHENSIVE APPLICATIONS OF SHAOLIN CHIN NA
CONFLICT COMMUNICATION
CROCODILE AND THE CRANE: A NOVEL
CUTTING SEASON: A XENON PEARL MARTIAL ARTS THRILLER
DAO DE JING
DAO IN ACTION
DEFENSIVE TACTICS
DESHI: A CONNOR BURKE MARTIAL ARTS THRILLER
DIRTY GROUND
DR. WU'S HEAD MASSAGE
DUKKHA HUNGRY GHOSTS
DUKKHA REVERB
DUKKHA, THE SUFFERING: AN EYE FOR AN EYE
DUKKHA UNLOADED
ENZAN: THE FAR MOUNTAIN, A CONNOR BURKE MARTIAL ARTS
  THRILLER
ESSENCE OF SHAOLIN WHITE CRANE
EVEN IF KILLS ME
EXPLORING TAI CHI
FACING VIOLENCE
FIGHT BACK
FIGHT LIKE A PHYSICIST
THE FIGHTER'S BODY
FIGHTER'S FACT BOOK
FIGHTER'S FACT BOOK 2
THE FIGHTING ARTS
FIGHTING THE PAIN RESISTANT ATTACKER
FIRST DEFENSE
FORCE DECISIONS: A CITIZENS GUIDE
FOX BORROWS THE TIGER'S AWE
INSIDE TAI CHI
THE JUDO ADVANTAGE
THE JUJI GATAME ENCYCLOPEDIA
KAGE: THE SHADOW, A CONNOR BURKE MARTIAL ARTS THRILLER
KARATE SCIENCE
KATA AND THE TRANSMISSION OF KNOWLEDGE
KRAV MAGA COMBATIVES
KRAV MAGA PROFESSIONAL TACTICS
KRAV MAGA WEAPON DEFENSES
LITTLE BLACK BOOK OF VIOLENCE
LIUHEBAFA FIVE CHARACTER SECRETS
MARTIAL ARTS ATHLETE
MARTIAL ARTS INSTRUCTION
MARTIAL WAY AND ITS VIRTUES
MASK OF THE KING
MEDITATIONS ON VIOLENCE
MERIDIAN QIGONG EXERCISES
MIND/BODY FITNESS
MINDFUL EXERCISE
THE MIND INSIDE TAI CHI
THE MIND INSIDE YANG STYLE TAI CHI CHUAN
MUGAI RYU
NATURAL HEALING WITH QIGONG
NORTHERN SHAOLIN SWORD, 2ND ED.
OKINAWA'S COMPLETE KARATE SYSTEM: ISSHIN RYU
THE PAIN-FREE BACK

PAIN-FREE JOINTS
POWER BODY
PRINCIPLES OF TRADITIONAL CHINESE MEDICINE
THE PROTECTOR ETHIC
QIGONG FOR HEALTH & MARTIAL ARTS 2ND ED.
QIGONG FOR LIVING
QIGONG FOR TREATING COMMON AILMENTS
QIGONG MASSAGE
QIGONG MEDITATION: EMBRYONIC BREATHING
QIGONG MEDITATION: SMALL CIRCULATION
QIGONG, THE SECRET OF YOUTH: DA MO'S CLASSICS
QUIET TEACHER: A XENON PEARL MARTIAL ARTS THRILLER
RAVEN'S WARRIOR
REDEMPTION
ROOT OF CHINESE QIGONG, 2ND ED.
SAMBO ENCYCLOPEDIA
SCALING FORCE
SELF-DEFENSE FOR WOMEN
SENSEI: A CONNOR BURKE MARTIAL ARTS THRILLER
SHIHAN TE: THE BUNKAI OF KATA
SHIN GI TAI: KARATE TRAINING FOR BODY, MIND, AND SPIRIT
SIMPLE CHINESE MEDICINE
SIMPLE QIGONG EXERCISES FOR HEALTH, 3RD ED.
SIMPLIFIED TAI CHI CHUAN, 2ND ED.
SOLO TRAINING
SOLO TRAINING 2
SUMO FOR MIXED MARTIAL ARTS
SUNRISE TAI CHI
SUNSET TAI CHI
SURVIVING ARMED ASSAULTS
TAE KWON DO: THE KOREAN MARTIAL ART
TAEKWONDO BLACK BELT POOMSAE
TAEKWONDO: A PATH TO EXCELLENCE
TAEKWONDO: ANCIENT WISDOM FOR THE MODERN WARRIOR
TAEKWONDO: DEFENSE AGAINST WEAPONS
TAEKWONDO: SPIRIT AND PRACTICE
TAO OF BIOENERGETICS
TAI CHI BALL QIGONG: FOR HEALTH AND MARTIAL ARTS
TAI CHI BALL WORKOUT FOR BEGINNERS
THE TAI CHI BOOK
TAI CHI CHIN NA: THE SEIZING ART OF TAI CHI CHUAN,
  2ND ED.
TAI CHI CHUAN CLASSICAL YANG STYLE, 2ND ED.
TAI CHI CHUAN MARTIAL POWER, 3RD ED.
TAI CHI CONNECTIONS
TAI CHI DYNAMICS
TAI CHI FOR DEPRESSION
TAI CHI IN 10 WEEKS
TAI CHI QIGONG, 3RD ED.
TAI CHI SECRETS OF THE ANCIENT MASTERS
TAI CHI SECRETS OF THE WU & LI STYLES
TAI CHI SECRETS OF THE WU STYLE
TAI CHI SECRETS OF THE YANG STYLE
TAI CHI SWORD: CLASSICAL YANG STYLE, 2ND ED.
TAI CHI SWORD FOR BEGINNERS
TAI CHI WALKING
TAIJIQUAN THEORY OF DR. YANG, JWING-MING
TAO OF BIOENERGETICS
TENGU: THE MOUNTAIN GOBLIN, A CONNOR BURKE MARTIAL ARTS
  THRILLER
TIMING IN THE FIGHTING ARTS
TRADITIONAL CHINESE HEALTH SECRETS
TRADITIONAL TAEKWONDO
TRAINING FOR SUDDEN VIOLENCE
TRUE WELLNESS
TRUE WELLNESS: THE MIND
THE WARRIOR'S MANIFESTO
WAY OF KATA
WAY OF KENDO AND KENJITSU
WAY OF SANCHIN KATA
WAY TO BLACK BELT
WESTERN HERBS FOR MARTIAL ARTISTS
WILD GOOSE QIGONG
WINNING FIGHTS
WISDOM'S WAY
XINGYIQUAN

DVDS FROM YMAA

ADVANCED PRACTICAL CHIN NA IN-DEPTH
ANALYSIS OF SHAOLIN CHIN NA
ATTACK THE ATTACK
BAGUA FOR BEGINNERS 1
BAGUA FOR BEGINNERS 2
BAGUAZHANG: EMEI BAGUAZHANG
BEGINNER QIGONG FOR WOMEN 1
BEGINNER QIGONG FOR WOMEN 2
BEGINNER TAI CHI FOR HEALTH
CHEN STYLE TAIJIQUAN
CHEN TAI CHI FOR BEGINNERS
CHIN NA IN-DEPTH COURSES 1—4
CHIN NA IN-DEPTH COURSES 5—8
CHIN NA IN-DEPTH COURSES 9—12
FACING VIOLENCE: 7 THINGS A MARTIAL ARTIST MUST KNOW
FIVE ANIMAL SPORTS
FIVE ELEMENTS ENERGY BALANCE
INFIGHTING
INTRODUCTION TO QI GONG FOR BEGINNERS
JOINT LOCKS
KNIFE DEFENSE: TRADITIONAL TECHNIQUES AGAINST A DAGGER
KUNG FU BODY CONDITIONING 1
KUNG FU BODY CONDITIONING 2
KUNG FU FOR KIDS
KUNG FU FOR TEENS
LOGIC OF VIOLENCE
MERIDIAN QIGONG
NEIGONG FOR MARTIAL ARTS
NORTHERN SHAOLIN SWORD : SAN CAI JIAN, KUN WU JIAN, QI MEN JIAN
QI GONG 30-DAY CHALLENGE
QI GONG FOR ANXIETY
QI GONG FOR ARMS, WRISTS, AND HANDS
QIGONG FOR BEGINNERS: FRAGRANCE
QI GONG FOR BETTER BREATHING
QI GONG FOR CANCER
QI GONG FOR ENERGY AND VITALITY
QI GONG FOR HEADACHES
QI GONG FOR HEALING
QI GONG FOR HEALTHY JOINTS
QI GONG FOR HIGH BLOOD PRESSURE
QIGONG FOR LONGEVITY
QI GONG FOR STRONG BONES
QI GONG FOR THE UPPER BACK AND NECK
QIGONG FOR WOMEN
QIGONG FOR WOMEN WITH DAISY LEE
QIGONG MASSAGE
QIGONG MINDFULNESS IN MOTION
QIGONG: 15 MINUTES TO HEALTH
SABER FUNDAMENTAL TRAINING
SAI TRAINING AND SEQUENCES
SANCHIN KATA: TRADITIONAL TRAINING FOR KARATE POWER
SCALING FORCE
SHAOLIN KUNG FU FUNDAMENTAL TRAINING: COURSES 1 & 2
SHAOLIN LONG FIST KUNG FU: ADVANCED SEQUENCES 1
SHAOLIN LONG FIST KUNG FU: ADVANCED SEQUENCES 2
SHAOLIN LONG FIST KUNG FU: BASIC SEQUENCES
SHAOLIN LONG FIST KUNG FU: INTERMEDIATE SEQUENCES
SHAOLIN SABER: BASIC SEQUENCES

SHAOLIN STAFF: BASIC SEQUENCES
SHAOLIN WHITE CRANE GONG FU BASIC TRAINING: COURSES 1 & 2
SHAOLIN WHITE CRANE GONG FU BASIC TRAINING: COURSES 3 & 4
SHUAI JIAO: KUNG FU WRESTLING
SIMPLE QIGONG EXERCISES FOR HEALTH
SIMPLE QIGONG EXERCISES FOR ARTHRITIS RELIEF
SIMPLE QIGONG EXERCISES FOR BACK PAIN RELIEF
SIMPLIFIED TAI CHI CHUAN: 24 & 48 POSTURES
SIMPLIFIED TAI CHI FOR BEGINNERS 48
SUNRISE TAI CHI
SUNSET TAI CHI
SWORD: FUNDAMENTAL TRAINING
TAEKWONDO KORYO POOMSAE
TAI CHI BALL QIGONG: COURSES 1 & 2
TAI CHI BALL QIGONG: COURSES 3 & 4
TAI CHI BALL WORKOUT FOR BEGINNERS
TAI CHI CHUAN CLASSICAL YANG STYLE
TAI CHI CONNECTIONS
TAI CHI ENERGY PATTERNS
TAI CHI FIGHTING SET
TAI CHI FIT: 24 FORM
TAI CHI FIT: FLOW
TAI CHI FIT: FUSION BAMBOO
TAI CHI FIT: FUSION FIRE
TAI CHI FIT: FUSION IRON
TAI CHI FIT IN PARADISE
TAI CHI FIT: OVER 50
TAI CHI FIT: STRENGTH
TAI CHI FIT: TO GO
TAI CHI FOR WOMEN
TAI CHI FUSION: FIRE
TAI CHI QIGONG
TAI CHI PUSHING HANDS: COURSES 1 & 2
TAI CHI PUSHING HANDS: COURSES 3 & 4
TAI CHI SWORD: CLASSICAL YANG STYLE
TAI CHI SWORD FOR BEGINNERS
TAI CHI SYMBOL: YIN YANG STICKING HANDS
TAIJI & SHAOLIN STAFF: FUNDAMENTAL TRAINING
TAIJI CHIN NA IN-DEPTH
TAIJI 37 POSTURES MARTIAL APPLICATIONS
TAIJI SABER CLASSICAL YANG STYLE
TAIJI WRESTLING
TRAINING FOR SUDDEN VIOLENCE
UNDERSTANDING QIGONG 1: WHAT IS QI? • HUMAN QI CIRCULATORY SYSTEM
UNDERSTANDING QIGONG 2: KEY POINTS • QIGONG BREATHING
UNDERSTANDING QIGONG 3: EMBRYONIC BREATHING
UNDERSTANDING QIGONG 4: FOUR SEASONS QIGONG
UNDERSTANDING QIGONG 5: SMALL CIRCULATION
UNDERSTANDING QIGONG 6: MARTIAL QIGONG BREATHING
WATER STYLE FOR BEGINNERS
WHITE CRANE HARD & SOFT QIGONG
YANG TAI CHI FOR BEGINNERSS
WUDANG KUNG FU: FUNDAMENTAL TRAINING
WUDANG SWORD
WUDANG TAIJIQUAN
XINGYIQUAN
YANG TAI CHI FOR BEGINNERS

more products available from . . .

YMAA Publication Center, Inc. 楊氏東方文化出版中心

1-800-669-8892 • info@ymaa.com • www.ymaa.com